175108

Topics in Environmental Physiology and Medicine

edited by Karl E. Schaefer

Man and Animals in Hot Environments

D. L. Ingram and L. E. Mount

Springer-Verlag New York Heidelberg Berlin
1975

D. L. Ingram
and
L. E. Mount

Agricultural Research Council
Institute of Animal Physiology
Babraham
Cambridge CB2 4AT
England

Library of Congress Cataloging in Publication Data

Ingram, Douglas Leslie, 1929–
  Man and animals in hot environments.

  (Topics in environmental physiology and medicine)
  Bibliography: p.
  Includes index.
  1. Heat—Physiological effect.   2.   Acclimatization.
3.   Adaptation (Physiology)   I.   Mount, Laurence Edward,
joint author.   II.   Title.
QP82.2.H4I53   596′.01′9162   74–32104

Printed in the United States of America.

ISBN 0-387-06865-1 Springer-Verlag New York Heidelberg Berlin
ISBN 3-540-06865-1 Springer-Verlag Berlin Heidelberg New York

Sometime too hot the eye of heaven shines
William Shakespeare

Preface

This book is an introduction to the physiological reactions of man and animals to hot environments. It is intended for those who already have some knowledge of physiology. The aim has been to bridge the gap between general texts on physiology and advanced books on environmental physiology that deal with the specific problems of particular regions or individual species. Advanced works of this kind are referred to in the text and given in the bibliography.

The bibliography is extensive, but in spite of the formidable literature we are still ignorant of many aspects of thermal physiology, and the species that have been studied in detail are only a small proportion of those that may usefully receive attention. Physiologists have often seemed to assume that all animals are similar to man, dogs, cats, and rats, but these species have been chosen for study on the basis of convenience and not because they are representative of animals as a whole. There is another basis on which the selection of species for study can be made, however, and that is their usefulness to man. Man is of obvious interest to himself and has been given a separate chapter, but in the chapters on animals emphasis has been placed, when possible, on those species that have been domesticated and on which man depends for food and labor.

Although we are responsible for any errors and mistakes of judgment, it is a pleasure to acknowledge the help of our colleagues who have read the manuscript and made useful criticisms. In particular, we wish to thank Dr. J. Bligh, Institute of Animal Physiology; Dr. H. J. Carlisle, University of California; Prof. O. G. Edholm, University of London; Dr. K. J. Collins, London School of Hygiene and Tropical Medicine; the late Dr. J. D. Findlay, Hannah Research Institute; Prof. J. L. Monteith, F.R.S., University of Nottingham; and Dr. G. C. Whittow, University of Hawaii. We also wish to make grateful acknowledgment to the many authors who have given permission for material to be reproduced, and to Mr. D. W. Butcher and the library staff of this institute for their help with the literature. We wish to thank Prof. R. D. Keynes, F.R.S., University of Cambridge, former Director of the institute, for his permission to undertake the work.

Finally we thank the following publishers, societies and journals for permission to use material: *American Journal of Medicine*; American Physiological Society; American Society of Agricultural Engineers; Baillière Tindall; Butterworths Ltd.; Cambridge University Press; Charles C Thomas; College of Agriculture, Columbia, Missouri;

Die Naturwissenschaften; Edward Arnold Ltd.; *Farm Mechanization and Buildings*; *Journal of Agricultural Science*; *Journal of Reproduction and Fertility*; Lea and Febiger; Masson et Cie, Paris; MacMillan Publishing Co., Inc.; National Academy of Science, U.S.; National Research Council of Canada; *Nature*, London; North Holland Publishing Co.; Oxford University Press; Pergamon Press; *Physiology and Behavior*; Poultry Science Association; Reinhold Publishing Co.; Research in Veterinary Science; Springer Verlag; The Ciba Foundation Ltd.; The Institute of Biology; *The Lancet*; The Physiological Society (G. B.); The Royal Society; University of Chicago Press; University of Rhodesia; *Verhandlungen der Deutschen Gesellschaft für Kreislaufforschung*; Waverly Press; and W. B. Saunders.

D. L. INGRAM
L. E. MOUNT

Contents

Adaptations to Hot Environments

CHAPTER 1

The Thermal Environment

Hot, Thermally Neutral, and Cold Environments

The deep body temperature of homeo-thermic animals is maintained within fairly narrow limits by elaborate thermoregulatory mechanisms. These rely on a large number of graded physiological, morpohological, and behavioral responses, which in turn depend on the thermal nature of the environment. The thermal characteristics of the environment are essentially air temperature, radiant temperatures (infrared and solar radiation), rate of air movement, humidity, wetting by precipitation or otherwise, and in certain cases the nature of the floor. These thermal characteristics determine the levels of heat exchange between animal and environment (Chapters 2 and 3).

The term "heat exchange" implies either heat loss from the animal to the environment or heat gain by the animal. In the cold, animals lose heat through channels that depend on a temperature gradient, that is, by radiation, convection, and conduction. These channels are often termed "sensible" because the loss of heat through them is a form of energy transfer that can be detected by the senses. Under hot conditions animals tend to gain heat through these channels and can lose heat to the environment only by evaporation either from the body surface (by sweating or by the evaporation of water other than sweat) or by panting (Chapters 3 and 4). In the cold, the primary problem for animals is conserving the heat they produce, an end achieved by insulative and behavioral adaptations. Under hot conditions, in contrast, the problem is one of heat dissipation by physiological and behavioral means (Chapters 4, 5, and 7). Between cold and hot lies an intermediate range in which animals find little difficulty in maintaining body temperature. This zone varies with species and the age and adaptation of the animal, and is related to the zone of thermal neutrality (Chapters 2 and 3) in which the rate of heat production is at a minimum.

Below a certain air temperature an increase in the rate of oxygen consumption occurs in homeothermic animals. This air temperature, which must be determined under given conditions as discussed below, is termed the "critical temperature." Below this point the environmental conditions can be described as "cold" because the animal must increase its metabolism in order to maintain thermal equilibrium. Immediately above the critical temperature there is a range of temperature over which oxygen consumption does not change. However, at some still higher air temperature the animal's body temperature begins to increase because heat cannot be lost fast enough. As a consequence of this increase in the temperature of the tissues, and because chemical reactions proceed faster at higher temperatures, oxygen consumption increases. The oxygen consumption curve for a hypothetical mammal is shown in Fig. 1–1.

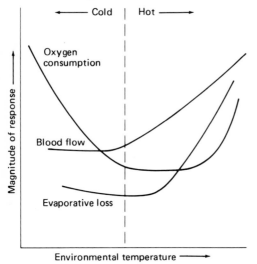

Fig. 1–1. Oxygen consumption curve for a hypothetical homeotherm. The terms "hot" and "cold" can be defined in terms of the animal's physiological responses to its environmental temperature.

The rate at which heat is lost through radiation, convection, and conduction can be modified by changes in the rate at which blood flows through the skin (Chapter 5). Variations in the rate of peripheral blood flow alter the tissue insulation between the core and the skin surface and the skin temperature. Below the critical temperature the rate of peripheral blood flow is very small. If the rate of peripheral blood flow is measured as the air temperature is increased (Fig. 1–1), both the flow and the skin temperature begin to increase near the critical temperature and heat loss is facilitated.

Below the critical temperature the loss of water by evaporation from the skin is small. As the environmental temperature rises above the critical level evaporative heat loss is increased (Chapter 4). As the temperature rises still further, sensible heat loss declines toward zero and the evaporative channel becomes the only effective route for heat loss.

In the idealized diagram of Fig. 1–1 there is a range of temperature over which oxygen consumption and evaporative heat loss remain at a minimum and only peripheral blood flow changes. Within this range of environmental conditions, thermal equilibrium can be maintained with a minimum expenditure of raw materials in the form of food and water, indicating a zone of minimal material demand. Some authors have recently suggested that the definition of thermal neutrality be restricted to this zone (Mount, 1974); the older definition of the term refers to the zone in which oxygen consumption is minimal. However, in some instances this wider zone can include temperatures at which sweating or panting occurs and that may therefore be considered as too hot for a strictly "neutral" zone. This matter is given further attention in Chapter 3.

It is most important to appreciate that in Fig. 1–1 environmental temperature has been represented as simply the air temperature as measured with a dry bulb thermometer. There is no indication that air movement, radiant temperature, or humidity are involved. If, however, the critical temperature is determined as air temperature in environments with different wind speeds, for example, the critical temperature is higher under more windy conditions than in still air. This is because convective heat transfer for a given air temperature is greater in a wind than in still air. Similarly, if the critical temperature is determined at constant air temperature but under different conditions of radiant heating, it is found that when the radiant temperature is high the critical temperature is reduced. To avoid this confusion it is usual to have the air movement as low as possible and to specify the critical temperature in an environment with the radiant temperature the same as the air temperature. The exact conditions should in any event be stated.

Even when the climatic conditions have been fixed, however, other factors in the environment can influence the critical air temperature; for example, the provision of straw bedding lowers the critical temperature because it enables the animal to increase the amount of external insulation. Two or more animals together can modify the effects of a fall in ambient temperature by huddling, and even a single animal can alter the surface area of its body available for radiant, convective, and conductive heat transfer simply by changing its posture.

There are several additional factors that can influence the effect of a given environment on an animal's physiological responses to temperature. Animals on a high level of food intake have a lower critical temperature than those on a low level (Chapter 3). Metabolism may be influenced by the animal's previous thermal history: the resting metabolism of an animal that has been exposed to heat for some days is lower than that of a control animal exposed to the cold. Prolonged exposure to a particular set of conditions also influences the endocrine system (Chapter 6). Seasonal changes often occur in the amount of external insulation so that the critical temperature is lower in the winter than in the summer. Such animals as mice that have been raised from birth in a hot environment grow longer tails and so have a greater surface area available for heat exchange. A further complication is that all measurements should be made under steady-state conditions, that is, when body temperature is not changing. If this condition is not met, then account must be taken of the heat that has been stored in the body or lost. In practice, the condition can only be met over short periods because body temperature tends to fluctuate rhythmically over a 24-hour period.

This combination of effects means that it is very difficult to make strict comparisons between animals even of the same species. What is a warm environment for one animal may be a cold one for another. This is certainly true for members of the same species but of different age, for example, newborn and mature pigs. Among species the differences may be very great indeed. The arctic fox in winter has a critical temperature below $-30°C$, whereas the laboratory rat's critical temperature is about $+28°C$. As a result a room at $10°C$ is "warm" for the fox and "cold" for the rat.

The reaction of animals and man to hot environments is discussed in Chapters 9 and 10. These discussions are limited, for the most part, to the climatic aspects of the environment, but it must be appreciated that both animals and man live in microenvironments that may be quite different from the surrounding macroenvironments. Man, especially, modifies his surroundings and may create a hot environment, such as a boiler room, in a temperate climate or he may, like the Eskimo, use clothes with a high insulation and so contrive to live in a subtropical microenvironment although the air temperature is below zero.

Development of Climatic Physiology

To a large extent the development and understanding of climatic physiology depended on progress in the physical sciences. As Mendelsohn's historical survey (1964) showed, the heat generated by animals has intrigued man since early times. However, until the development of measuring instruments an understanding of the problems involved was not possible. For example, the idea that the heart was the seat of an innate burning heat was held for hundreds of years before the temperature in the heart of an animal was measured with a mercury-in-glass thermometer in the seventeenth century. There still remained a confusion over the distinction between temperature and quantity of heat, a confusion (it might be added) that has sometimes occurred even today.

Some idea of early investigations in climatic physiology can be gained from reading two papers by Blagden (1774, 1775), which must be among the first written on the effects of a hot environment on man and animals. These reports include a much-quoted reference to experiments in which it was demonstrated that a man or a dog could survive in a hot room for the length of time it took a piece of meat exposed to the same environment to be cooked. Some extracts of the first paper are reproduced below (by permission of The Royal Society), but the originals are worth reading in full, both for the style and for the content.

Experiments and Observations
in an Heated Room
By Charles Blagden, M.D., F.R.S.
Redde Feb 16 1774

About the middle of January several gentlemen and myself received an invitation from Dr. George Fordyce, to observe the effects of air heated to a much higher degree than it was formerly thought any living creature could bear. We all rejoiced at the opportunity of being convinced, by our own experience, of the wonderful power with which the animal body is endued, of resisting an heat vastly greater than its own temperature; and our curiosity was not a little excited to observe the circumstances attending this remarkable power.

The second paper was read more than a year later and involved temperatures up to 260°F. The use of the terms "temperature" and "heat" in these papers suggests very strongly that at this time the distinction of meaning between them was not fully appreciated; for example, "Many repeated trials in successively higher degrees of heat, gave still more remarkable proofs of our resisting power" and again "pure water was heated to 140°F of the thermometer, whilst that with the wax had acquired an heat of 152°F," or "the actual heat of my body, tried under my tongue, and by applying closely the thermometer to my skin, was 98°F, about a degree higher than its ordinary temperature."

From other passages it is clear that a number of key observations have been made in these studies. For example, Blagden suffers more effect from the first exposure than from those reported in the second study, and he records that the first experiments have been made in the evening after a heavy meal. He also comments that the heat is more readily endured when the air is still and suggests that this is because air in contact with the body is cooled. In other words, he appreciates the effects of a boundary layer of air. In a footnote there is an interesting observation on evaporative cooling in amphibia.

> I applied a thermometer, in a hot summmer day, to the belly of a frog, and found the quicksilver sink several degrees: a rude experiment indeed, but serving to confirm the general fact, that the living body possesses a power of resisting the communication of heat.

However, it is not very clear whether Blagden fully appreciates the effects of evaporation because he seems to have believed that man's ability to withstand temperatures above body temperature is not entirely due to the vaporization of water.

In the following chapters the present state of knowledge about the reactions of man and animals to hot environments will be examined.

CHAPTER 2

Heat Exchange between Animal and Environment

Metabolic Heat and Its Dissipation

As a result of its metabolic activity, an animal produces heat. The rate at which heat is produced bears a direct relation to the metabolic rate measured as oxygen consumption. For this reason the two rates are often considered as relating to the same quantity and as being interchangeable, provided the animal is not doing external work. Although "metabolic rate" and "heat production" may have the same meaning, they are not necessarily of the same magnitude as heat loss. The rate of heat loss from an animal is determined by the rate of heat production and the rate at which heat is being lost from or stored in the body as the result of changes in the temperatures of its parts:

$$M = H + S \qquad (2\text{--}1)$$

where M = rate of heat production, or metabolic rate

H = rate of heat loss

S = rate of change of stored heat

M is always positive because it represents a collection of reactions of net exothermic value. S may be positive or negative; it is positive when the mean body temperature is rising and heat is being stored in the body and it is negative when the mean body temperature is falling. H is much more commonly positive than negative because the animal's net requirement is the dissipation of metabolic heat production. However, H can be negative, as for example in the rewarming following hypothermia or under conditions that induce hyperthermia, when there is a large positive storage rate derived from environmental heating. Under these conditions the environment acts as a heat source and not as a heat sink for the animal's metabolic heat. H is given by:

$$H = H_R + H_C + H_D + H_E \qquad (2\text{--}2)$$

where H_R = radiant heat loss

H_C = conductive heat loss

H_D = conductive heat loss

H_E = evaporative heat loss

H_R, H_C, and H_D may individually or collectively be positive (net heat loss from the animal, with the environment as a heat sink) or negative (net heat gain, with the environment as a heat source), depending on the temperature relations between animal and environment. H_E is nearly always positive, although under extreme conditions there may be net condensation of water vapor on an animal placed in an environment with a dewpoint above the skin temperature.

The relation among the production, loss, and storage of heat in the organism indicates the manner in which heat from metabolic processes is dissipated. Without loss to the environment, heat can be stored temporarily in the body but this mechanism is limited by the entailed rise in body temperature. For example, if a 70-kg man has a thermal capacity of 3.47 kJ kg^{-1} °C^{-1} (Burton and Edholm, 1955), a mean rise in body temperature of 1°C absorbs 70 × 3.47 = 242.9 kJ, which represents approximately 35 minutes of resting heat production. Heat is stored when the organism is exposed to high environmental temperatures that change heat loss into a heat gain from the environment, so that H becomes negative. S then becomes positive, both because of metabolic heat production and because of heat gained from the environment. This situation occurs in the camel during the daytime, when it is exposed to high temperatures. The animal's body temperature rises several degrees during the day and then falls during the succeeding night.

The subject of thermal capacity and body heat content in man has been discussed by Minard (1970). The difference between heat production and heat loss represents the change in heat content. When this change is divided by the thermal capacity, the change in mean body temperature is derived. A value of 3.47 kJ kg^{-1} °C^{-1}, which has been assumed for man for some time, lies between the extremes of 1.88 for fat and 4.18 for water; the value for lean flesh has been determined as 3.47. A closer approximation to the true value may therefore be based on the fat content of the subject. A higher fat content leads to a lower specific heat and a lower fat content to a higher specific heat. In practice, however, 3.47 kJ kg^{-1} °C^{-1} is commonly used.

Body Temperature

The implication of thermoregulation in the homeotherm is that body temperature is controlled, by processes of heat production and heat loss, at a stable level that is approximately maintained in spite of fluctuations in the environment. It is, in fact, the deep body temperature that is the controlled quantity; peripheral tissue temperatures vary considerably, depending on ambient conditions. The proportion of the body at the core temperature of 37°C in man is expanded under warm conditions, with a high skin temperature, and contracted in the cold, with a low skin temperature (Fig. 2–1). More ex-

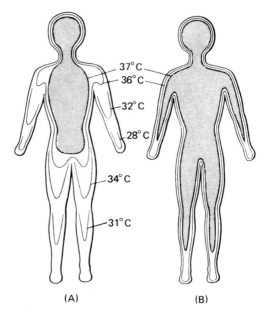

Fig. 2–1. Diagrammatic isotherms in the human body exposed to cold (A) and warm (B) conditions. The core of deep body temperature (shaded) shrinks in the cold, leaving a peripheral shell of cooler tissue (Aschoff and Wever, 1958).

treme temperature variations within the organism occur in other animals, examples being the very low foot temperature in the herring gull exposed to cold and the low skin temperature in the pig raised in a cold environment (Irving, 1964). It follows that there is no single body temperature and that the term "homeotherm" applies essentially to the maintenance of a stable core temperature. If the skin temperature is held at a given level by the animal's metabolic responses and if the metabolizing tissues are also deep in the animal, the deep body temperature varies considerably for the following reasons. If the environment becomes cooler, so that heat loss from the animal increases, the rate of heat production must increase if the skin temperature is to remain constant. Because the animal's thermal insulation between its core and periphery is finite, and although sometimes very slight is never zero, the increased rate of heat production leads to a rise in the temperature difference between core and periphery. In practice, the only situations in which surface temperature control leads to stable deep temperature control are the cases of a highly conducting, centrally heated object, such as a metal sphere containing an electric heater, and of forced convection in a fluid, as in a rapidly stirred water bath containing a heater.

Although the core temperature is stable in the sense that it does not fluctuate rapidly when the environment changes, it is not constant. It varies with time of day, activity and environmental conditions. The actual manner in which the body temperature is controlled in the homeotherm has been the subject of continuing extensive discussion and many explanations have been put forward. Accounts of the experimental evidence on which some of the hypotheses and models have been based can be found in a number of reviews (Hardy, 1961; Bligh, 1966).

Variations in temperature in different parts of the organism are associated with variations in heat storage. The practical implication of this in measuring heat loss from an animal is that heat loss is increased or decreased by changes in heat storage. The direct measurement of heat loss is therefore limited as an indication of metabolic rate. Burton (1935) has derived the mean body temperature for man as $0.65 \, T_R + 0.35 \, T_S$, where T_R is the rectal temperature and T_S is the mean skin temperature. He bases his calculations on 54 percent of the body volume lying within 25 mm of the body surface. Although T_S contributes only one-third of the mean body temperature, its variation is usually much greater than that of T_R.

Poikilotherm and Homeotherm

In poikilotherms, the body temperature tends to follow the environmental temperature because the resting level of heat production is very low and because there is no autonomic thermoregulatory system of the type existing in mammals and birds. This does not mean that the body temperature is always the same as the environmental temperature. The body temperature in insects rises when they become active, and this rise permits a higher level of metabolism than can occur at the lower level. This is an example of activity producing a difference between body and environmental temperatures in a poikilotherm. In certain lizards, a relatively stable body temperature can be produced by the animal moving between sun and shade. This use of environmental diversity to give a measure of thermoregulation is clearly itself environment-dependent, whereas the example of the active insect shows how a gradient can be maintained between body and environment by metabolic means.

Such poikilothermic regulations differ from those in the homeotherm both in the range of mechanisms at the animal's disposal and in the ways in which these are integrated functionally. Both the metabolic rate and the vasomotor and pilomotor effects on the rate of heat loss in the homeotherm are governed centrally. Effects of peripheral origin involve behavioral adjustments, including activity and posture. The net result in the homeotherm is the maintenance of a relatively stable deep body temperature in spite of fluctuations in environmental temperature. Stability, although limited in extent and duration, also occurs in the poikilotherm, but the built-in autonomic mechanism is absent.

The metabolic rate in the poikilotherm increases as body temperature increases, according to the van't Hoff effect, over the whole temperature range (Fuhrman and Fuhrman, 1959). The Q_{10} is the factor by which the velocity of a reaction is multiplied by a rise in temperature of $10°C$ and is given by the equation:

$$Q_{10} = \left(\frac{K_2}{K_1}\right)^{10/(T_2-T_1)} \qquad (2-3)$$

where K_1 and K_2 are velocity constants corresponding to temperatures T_1 and T_2. When, as often occurs, the rate of reaction is doubled by a rise of $10°C$, $Q_{10} = 2$. The homeotherm, in contrast, shows a relation between its body temperature and metabolic rate only at the extremes of cold and heat, where the body temperature is falling or rising (Graham et al., 1959; Mount, 1968a). At intermediate temperatures the body temperature is maintained at a steady level by variations in metabolic rate and thermal insulation that lead to greater or lesser heat losses, depending on whether the environmental temperature is lower or higher.

The homeotherm characteristically produces considerable heat and the minimum production under warm conditions is in excess of the requirement for thermoregulation. The considerable resting heat production of the homeotherm, compared with that of the poikilotherm, can be exemplified by a comparison of rodents and lizards in the desert. The metabolic rate of the desert rodent is about seven times that of the desert iguana at an environmental temperature of $37°C$, when the iguana's deep body temperature is similar to that of the rodent (Schmidt-Nielsen, 1964).

When the environmental temperature continues to rise, the metabolic rate in the homeotherm also eventually begins to rise, as does body temperature. The homeotherm is then behaving more like a poikilotherm in that its heat production is following the body temperature, which itself is following the environmental temperature. The animal is now outside the range within which it can control its body temperature, and unless it is removed to cooler conditions it dies in hyperthermia. A corresponding situation occurs when the environment is so cold that the animal's maximal metabolic response does not maintain body temperature. The metabolic rate and body temperature then decline together and the animal dies in hypothermia.

Heat Flow

The maintenance of a relatively stable core temperature in an organism exposed to a fluctuating environment presupposes some form of control of the flow of heat between the organism and its environment. It is apparent that a higher rate of heat production in a body can produce a higher body temperature. In addition, increased thermal insulation allows the temperature to rise although the rate of production of heat may remain constant. The homeotherm has control over both heat production and insulation and consequently exhibits a pattern of interrelation between heat flow, body–environment temperature difference, and thermal insulation. The modes of heat transfer between organism and environment are examined in this chapter and thermal insulation is considered in Chapter 3.

In most circumstances, the rate at which heat is lost or gained by a body is almost exactly proportional to the temperature difference between the body's surface and the environment. This relation is often described in terms of Newton's law of cooling, but this law, as it names implies, is primarily concerned with the rate of change of the temperature of the body. In an animal at equilibrium, cooling is not taking place although there is heat flow. It is therefore more appropriate to consider heat flow rather than cooling (Kleiber, 1961).

Heat flow is proportional to the temperature gradient and to the thermal conductance of the medium through which the heat is passing. This is a statement of Fourier's law, which may be expressed as:

$$H = \lambda \frac{A}{L}(T_1 - T_2) \qquad (2\text{--}4)$$

where H = rate of heat flow
   A = surface area
   L = thickness of medium through which heat is passing
   λ = thermal conductivity of medium
$T_1 - T_2$ = temperature difference across the medium

This can be rewritten in a form corresponding to Ohm's law for the flow of electricity:

$$H = A \frac{(T_1 - T_2)}{R} \qquad (2\text{--}5)$$

where $R = L/\lambda$
   = resistance to heat flow per unit cross-sectional area

In this instance, R can be defined as the "specific insulation," which is the insulation per unit area, a concept that can be applied to the thermal insulation between an animal's core and the environment. The reciprocal of the specific insulation is the thermal conductance, C:

$$H = AC(T_1 - T_2) \qquad (2\text{--}6)$$

The problem for the homeotherm under hot conditions is dissipating the heat it produces. The two modes of heat transfer through which heat dissipation can take place are the sensible and the evaporative. The term "sensible" is used here to indicate a mode of heat transfer that depends on a temperature gradient. It includes heat flow through radiation, convection, and conduction. Evaporative transfer, however, does not necessarily depend on a temperature gradient. It depends instead on the heat that is taken up by water when it changes from the liquid to the vapor state. Its particular significance is that loss of heat can still take place by this means even when the surroundings are at a higher temperature than the animal.

Sensible Heat Transfer

Each mode of sensible heat transfer depends primarily on the difference between the animal's surface temperature and the corresponding environmental temperature. The corresponding environmental temperatures are the mean radiant temperature, the air temperature, and the floor temperature, for radiative, convective, and conductive heat transfer, respectively. The magnitude of the heat flow through each channel also depends on additional factors, which are given in Table 2–1.

Radiation

Heat exchange by radiation in animals is conveniently considered in two parts. The first part deals with exchange when radiation from the surroundings is all "long wave," that is, emitted by surfaces at a range of temperatures extending downward from several hundred degrees centigrade. Long-wave radiation covers a range of wavelengths that has a maximum energy per unit wavelength occurring at a wavelength λ_{max}, which de-

Table 2–1   Factors that Influence the Different Modes of Heat Transfer between Organism and Environment

Mode of transfer	Animal characteristics	Environment characteristics
Radiant	Mean radiant temperature of surface; effective radiating area; reflectivity and emissivity	Mean radiant temperature; solar radiation and reflectivity of surroundings
Convective	Surface temperature; effective convective area; radius of curvature and surface type	Air temperature; air velocity and direction
Conductive	Surface temperature; effective contact area	Floor temperature; thermal conductivity and thermal capacity of solid material
Evaporative	Surface temperature; percentage wetted area; site of evaporation relative to skin surface	Humidity; air velocity and direction

creases as the temperature increases. The relation is given by Wien's displacement law (Jakob, 1949; Monteith, 1973), which states that $\lambda_{max} = 2897/T$ μm, where T is the absolute temperature. For a skin temperature of 30°C, λ_{max} is therefore 2897/303 = 9.6 μm; for 35°C it is 9.4 μm.

The second part of radiant exchange includes the effects of shorter wavelengths; that is, solar radiation, including the visible spectrum and the ultraviolet. Figure 2–2

shows the natural division that occurs between long-wave and short-wave radiant flux in the wavelength region between 2 and 3 μm.

An important feature of long-wave radiation is that it is transmitted by very few substances which are transparent to the shorter wavelengths of the visible spectrum. A common practical example of this is the horticultural greenhouse. Although the main effect of a greenhouse is to decrease con-

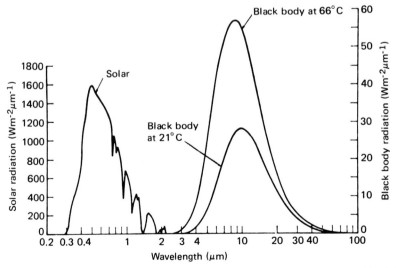

Fig. 2–2. Solar radiation at the ground for a zenith sun and radiation from black bodies at 21°C and 66°C (Bond et al., 1967, *Trans. Am. Soc. Agric. Engrs.* **10**: 622).

vective loss, there is also an effect on radiation balance. Glass allows the passage of the shorter wavelengths of radiation from the sun and sky, so that solar energy enters the house and warms it. The warm surfaces inside the house reradiate heat at the much longer wavelengths produced by their temperatures. Glass is opaque to these long wavelengths, so the direct radiation from objects inside the house is prevented from leaving it and contributes to the rise in inside temperature.

Another such situation occurs in hospital incubators for babies, because the Perspex (polymethyl methacrylate) of which they are made is also opaque to long-wave radiation. The consequences for the baby's thermal environment have been investigated by Hey and Mount (1967). Radiant heat exchange takes place between the baby and the inner surface of the Perspex wall and the mattress on which the baby lies. The temperature of the incubator wall therefore becomes important in determining the baby's radiant heat loss, because the wall occupies the major part of the solid angle subtended at the baby. The temperature of the inner surface of the wall is approximately halfway between the temperatures of the incubator air and the room air. Therefore, in a cool room the baby's radiant heat loss can be

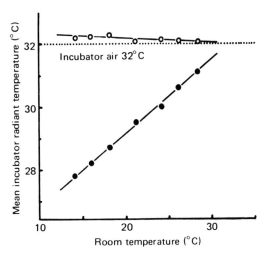

Fig. 2–3. The effect of room temperature on the mean radiant temperature within an incubator, with (○) and without (●) an internal shield at the temperature of the incubator air (Hey and Mount, 1966, *Lancet* **ii:** 202).

considerable. A thin Perspex shield placed between the baby and the wall reduces this loss, because the shield tends toward the temperature of the incubator air. As the shield is opaque to long-wave radiation from the baby, it creates a radiant environment warmer than the incubator wall (Fig. 2–3).

Polyethylene is one of the few substances that transmit the long infrared waves. In Fig. 2–4 the percentage transmittance of

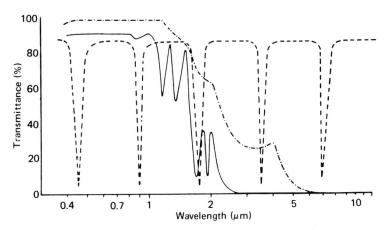

Fig. 2–4. The percentage transmittance of polyethylene, glass, and Perspex for radiation extending from the visible spectrum into the infrared (partly diagrammatic, for clarity). (– – –) 70-μm polyethylene, (— · —) 1-mm glass, (——) 6-mm Perspex (Mount, 1968a).

glass, Perspex, and polyethylene sheet are given in relation to wavelength. Glass and Perspex transmittance fall toward zero as the wavelength increases beyond 2–5 μm. In contrast, the transmittance of polyethylene remains high, with sharp troughs recurring at regular wavelength intervals because of the interference pattern associated with the CH_2 grouping in the molecule. If polyethylene is used instead of glass in making a greenhouse, the advantage that glass confers on preventing direct long-wave radiant heat loss from inside is not retained. The value of the polyethylene, in common with glass, then, is that it decreases heat loss by convection. In addition, any water droplets on the polyethylene markedly reduce its long-wave transmittance, because in the long-wave spectrum beyond 3 μm the absorptivity and emissivity of water are both about 0.995 (Monteith, 1973).

For the radiant heat emitted by skin, transmittance is at a minimum through glass and Perspex but is high through polyethylene. Polyethylene's property of transmitting such long-wave radiation has been used in shielding a radiometer (Funk, 1959), in experiments on the radiation cooling of dairy cattle carried out by Shanklin and Stewart (1958), and in the determination of the radiant heat exchange of the newborn pig (Mount, 1964a).

The factors involved in heat exchange by radiation are made explicit by the Stefan-Boltzmann law for total radiation from a perfectly black body:

$$H_R = \sigma A T^4 \qquad (2\text{--}7)$$

where H_R = rate of emission of radiation by a surface, W

σ = the Stefan-Boltzmann constant, 5.67 $\times 10^{-8}$ Wm^{-2} °K^{-4}

A = effective radiating area of body, m^2

T = absolute temperature of the radiating surface, °K

This is the radiation emitted by a given body, which depends on the fourth power of the absolute temperature T. What is required in practice, however, is the net radi-

ant exchange, which is the difference between the radiant energy leaving the body and the radiant energy entering it from the environment. An oft-quoted expression for the net radiant exchange is given by Hardy (1949):

$$H = \sigma e_1 e_2 A (T_1^4 - T_2^4) \qquad (2\text{--}8)$$

where e_1 and e_2 = the emissivities of the surfaces of the body and the surroundings

T_1 and T_2 = the absolute temperatures of the body and the surroundings

Emissivity has a maximum value of unity. This is the value for a perfectly black, opaque body, which reflects none of the incident radiation but absorbs all of it. An opaque perfect reflector, in contrast, has an emissivity of zero. It reflects all incident radiation and absorbs none of it. Such bodies do not exist in nature, although a matt black surface approaches a perfectly black surface in having an emissivity between 0.95 and 1.0. A nearly perfectly black surface is produced by a hollow enclosure with only a small opening; the opening itself then acts as a surface of absorptivity = emissivity = 1. The proof of this is given by Jakob (1949). An opaque body that absorbs much radiation reflects little, and vice versa. Absorptivity plus reflectivity equals unity, and absorptivity equals emissivity.

Emissivity varies with the wavelength of the radiation used. Figure 2–5 shows the variation in reflection power (and consequently the emissivity) of human skin when the wavelength of radiation is varied. The measurement of emissivity of skin has been discussed by Mitchell (1970). For wavelengths longer than 5 μm the emissivity of skin is close to unity, and this is true for most natural surfaces at this wavelength (e.g., vegetation, soil, water). The emissivity of white paint is as high as that of lamp black for long wavelengths, whereas white paint reflects to a large degree the shorter wavelengths characteristic of solar radiation. Polished metals have low long-wave emissivities and consequently high reflectivities.

Equation (2–8) is a satisfactory approximation provided that the emissivities e_1 and e_2 are both close to unity. As they fall below unity, however, the error involved in computing the radiant exchange increases, not only because of emissivity but also because a term involving the areas of the body and its surroundings becomes significant. To avoid these errors, it is necessary to use a more comprehensive equation than Eq. (2–8), and this requirement is met by Christiansen's equation (Jakob, 1957):

$$H_R = \frac{1}{1 + e_1(1/e_2 - 1) \, A_1/A_2} \cdot$$
$$e_1\sigma A_1(T_1^4 - T_2^4) \qquad (2–9)$$

where A_1 and A_2 refer to the effective radiating areas of the inner body and of the enclosure, respectively. This may be rewritten

$$H_R = F\sigma A_1(T_1^4 - T_2^4) \qquad (2–10)$$

where F is termed the radiative interchange factor and is defined by Eqs. (2–9) and (2–10). The factor allows for both the configuration and the emissivities of the surfaces. For long concentric cylinders, in which the areas of the end sections are insignificant compared with the areas of the curved surfaces, the ratio of areas is:

$$\frac{A_1}{A_2} = \frac{2\pi r_1}{2\pi r_2} = \frac{r_1}{r_2}$$

and for concentric spheres it is:

$$\frac{A_1}{A_2} = \frac{\pi r_1^2}{\pi r_2^2} = \frac{r_1^2}{r_2^2}$$

(see McGuire, 1953, and Monteith, 1973, for discussions of radiation geometry).

What is important in experiments in which the heat exchange of an animal within an enclosure is considered is that F, the radiative interchange factor, can be determined for a given situation without reference to the constitution of the factor, that is, whether it should be represented as (e_1e_2) or whether it should take the more precise form shown in Eq. (2–9). The chief disadvantage of this method is that any change in emissivity of the surface of either the animal or the enclosure may not be recognized and so causes error. However, the most probable change in long-wave emissivity is that caused by dust or other particulate matter, which raises the emissivity toward unity. In the long-wave spectrum relevant to the emission of heat from an animal's skin, the emissivity is already close to unity (Fig. 2–5), so any error caused by dust arises

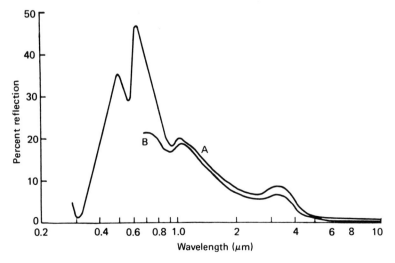

Fig. 2–5. The reflecting power of white (curve A) and Negro (curve B) skin over a range of wavelengths of radiation extending from the ultraviolet into the infrared (Hardy, 1949).

only in a polished enclosure. Where the emissivity e_2 of the enclosure surface approaches unity, the value for F given by Eqs. (2–9) and (2–10) tends toward e_1. Further discussion of radiant exchange is given elsewhere (Mount, 1968a; Monteith, 1973).

Convection

Whereas radiant heat exchange depends on the radiant temperature and effective radiating area and emissivity, heat exchange by convection depends on the surface temperature of the body; its shape, surface characteristics, and size; and the air temperature and the air movement rate that impinge upon it (see Table 2–1).

The basis of convective heat exchange has been discussed by Mitchell (1974). It depends on the redistribution of molecules within a fluid, as distinct from the conduction of heat, in which there is no actual translocation of molecules. Natural or free convection occurs because a temperature difference in a fluid gives rise to buoyancy forces. The way in which air rises after being warmed by a hot body is an example. "Forced convection" implies that the fluid movement takes place not because of temperature gradients but as the result of an external force moving the fluid. An example is cooling by air blown by a fan. In nearly still air a boundary layer forms on the surface of an object. It is this layer that produces most of the thermal insulation across a thin wall the substance of which has a high thermal conductivity. Figure 2–6 shows the temperature gradients across the Perspex wall of an incubator and demonstrates that the temperature change is nearly all in the boundary layers. Movement of the surface increases convective heat exchange considerably by disrupting the boundary layer. Increasing wind speed has the same effect. The nature of the surface of the body, that is, whether it is smooth or indented, naked or

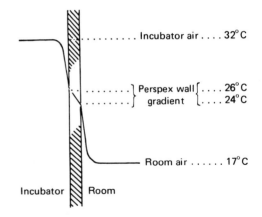

Fig. 2–6. Temperature gradients across the Perspex wall of a heated incubator. The thickness of the boundary layers, indicated by the sharp changes in temperature, is not drawn to scale (Hey and Mount, 1966).

coated, has a considerable effect on convective exchange. The size also has an effect; the smaller the radius of a part, the greater the convective heat loss per unit area for a given body–ambient temperature difference. These effects can be combined to give a "characteristic dimension" for the object in question. Hardy (1949), for example, points out that the adult human body behaves as a cylinder 7 cm in diameter, or a sphere 15 cm in diameter, if everything but convection is neglected.

Conduction

Compared with the information available on other channels of heat exchange, there is little on heat exchange by conduction in animals. In addition to the temperature of the floor, the thermal conductance and thermal capacity of the material of which the floor is composed are the environmental factors that determine the rate at which heat flows across the contact area with the animal. The relative effects of conductance and capacity can be demonstrated by the case of a young pig lying on a cement floor that has insulation built in beneath the top layer, a common arrangement in animal husbandry. The top layer itself has a relatively large thermal capacity and, if it is cold, heat flows from the animal for some considerable time before a steady state is reached. From this point on the underlying insulation becomes effective in reducing further heat flow. If the animal changes its position, it must warm succeeding fresh areas of floor. Therefore, it is the thermal capacity of the top layer that determines the floor's biologically important thermal characteristics, the lower layer of insulation being relatively ineffective.

Heat Loss to Ingesta

A small quantity of heat is also transferred to ingested food and water. At high environmental temperatures the voluntary intake of water is normally larger than under colder conditions. As an example, in calorimetric experiments at high temperatures, sheep take in quantities of water that are much greater than those required for urinary excretion and the animal's relatively small evaporative loss. In fact, sheep drink most frequently 1–2 hours after feeding, coincid-

ing with the maximum effect of the heat increment of feeding. The heat of warming both food and water to body temperature amounts to 2–3 W, representing about 3 percent of the total loss required to balance a heat production of the order of 100 W (Blaxter et al., 1959a). The heat lost by the pig in warming ingested water to body temperature also amounts to about 3 percent of the total heat loss (Mount, 1968a). In both animals, the quantity of water drunk under hot conditions considerably exceeds urinary and evaporative requirements.

Magnitude of Sensible Heat Transfer

As the environmental temperature rises, sensible heat transfer decreases. As the critical temperature is approached, however, the animal's skin temperature rises owing to vasodilatation, so that the rate at which the temperature difference between animal and environment decreases is slowed down. The result is that loss of sensible heat continues at a higher environmental temperature than is otherwise the case, as illustrated in Fig. 2–7. The heat loss referred to in the diagram is that by radiation and convection

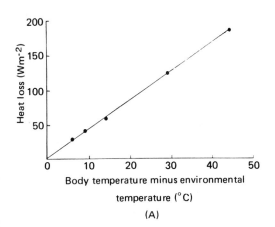

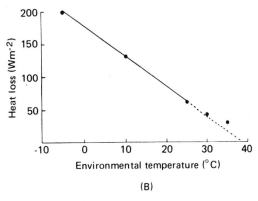

Fig. 2–7. (A) The relation between heat loss from the pig and the temperature difference between the body and the environment. (B) The relation between heat loss and environmental temperature (Ingram, 1964b).

from the flank of a young pig, measured by a heat-flow disk on the animal's surface.

At the higher temperatures, heat loss is higher than predicted by the broken straight line extrapolated from the points obtained at the lower temperatures. This disparity is associated with a rise in the pig's skin temperature. Clearly, however, this effect cannot be extended indefinitely as a mechanism compatible with life, for the animal's lethal temperature limit is soon reached. In practice, the rising environmental temperature overtakes the skin temperature, so that the gradient becomes reversed. Heat then passes from the environment to the animal, and the animal is consequently subjected to an environmental heat load in addition to its metabolic heat production. It is possible for an animal in this situation to lose through other channels as much sensible heat as the combined total of what it gains and produces. For example, the animal may lie on a cool floor to which heat is lost by conduction, or one aspect of the animal may be exposed to a low radiant temperature. When the net sensible heat exchange becomes zero, the only means of dissipating additional heat is by evaporative heat loss.

Evaporative Heat Transfer

During the rise of environmental temperature, evaporative loss increases before the environmental temperature reaches the surface temperature and, depending on the species, at a variable interval before hyperthermia ensues. In some species, notably man, environmental temperatures considerably above the deep body temperature can be tolerated because of the considerable ability to sweat. Consequently, large quantities of heat can be dissipated through the channel of evaporative loss, so that body temperature is regulated even under a relatively large heat load.

The basic quantity of heat involved in evaporative transfer is the latent heat of vaporization of water, a quantity that decreases from 2501 J/gm at 0°C to 2406 J/gm at 40°C. The factors influencing evaporative heat transfer are given in Table 2–1. The skin–ambient vapor pressure difference bears a relation to evaporative heat transfer similar to that which the skin–ambient temperature difference bears to sensible heat transfer. It is the difference in vapor pressure that constitutes the driving force for vaporization. The vapor pressure gives a measure of absolute humidity, as opposed to relative humidity, which gives a measure of that proportion of the saturation vapor pressure represented by the water vapor already present. When the water vapor pressure remains constant, the relative humidity falls as the temperature rises, because at higher temperatures the saturation vapor pressure is higher. For example, at 20°C, at the saturation vapor pressure of 23.3 mbar, the relative humidity is 100 percent; the vapor pressure is 11.7 mbar for 50 percent relative humidity. At 30°C, however, the saturation vapor pressure is 42.0 mbar and a vapor pressure of 23.3 mbar gives a relative humidity of only 55 percent and 11.7 mbar gives only 28 percent.

When liquid water is exposed in a closed volume at a given temperature, water vapor is formed and the vapor pressure rises until the saturation pressure for that particular temperature is reached. At that point, there is no further net formation of water vapor because the liquid and gaseous phases are in equilibrium. As the temperature rises, the saturation vapor pressure rises, and the equilibrium shifts with the net formation of more water vapor. The formation of water vapor and its equilibrium with liquid water is independent of the presence of air or other gases. It is not, in fact, the air that becomes saturated or that takes up water vapor. Instead, it is the quantity of water vapor per unit volume of space that is significant. Normally, however, it is the temperature of the air that is referred to in relation to humidity, and it is this which has given rise to the impression of the air as a sponge for water vapor, an impression that is quite erroneous. Water vapor exists as a gas and conforms to the gas laws with the limitations applicable to other gases. It is therefore not strictly appropriate to refer to the "relative humidity of the air" or to air being saturated; rather, the relative humidity and saturation should be considered only in relation to the amount of water vapor present. It is nonetheless convenient to consider air as the vehicle for water vapor, particularly when dealing with mass transport. The reason for this is the need to measure total gas movement, that is, air plus water vapor, and the practical consequence is to consider the amount of water vapor present as a proportion of the maximum that could be present. In general usage, therefore, one speaks of the relative humidity and the water-vapor carrying ability of the air (Goodman, 1944).

Figure 2–8, a psychrometric chart, gives the relation between temperature and water vapor pressure. The inset diagram on the chart shows the relation between the dry bulb (DB) and wet bulb (WB) temperatures, the relative humidity, the dew points, and the vapor pressure. "Dry bulb" is the term used to describe the temperature of the air obtained by a thermometer or thermocouple in the usual way, but it is essential that the sensing element be dry. If it is completely covered with a film of water, the "wet bulb" reading is obtained. This is lower than the dry bulb, the depression being caused by the evaporation of the water and consequent loss of heat from the bulb. The extent of the "wet bulb depression," as it is sometimes called, depends on the temperature and the ambient humidity. At low humidities, evaporation from the wet bulb occurs rapidly and the depression is large, whereas at high humidities evaporation is less and the wet bulb reading is closer to the dry bulb. There are many different designs of wet bulb equipment, some simple and some more complicated. The choice of particular apparatus depends on

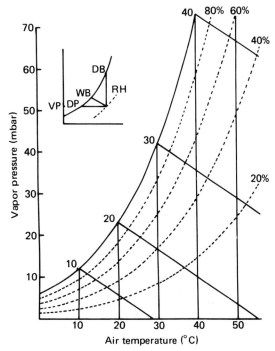

Fig. 2–8. Psychrometric chart relating dry (DB) and wet bulb (WB) temperatures to vapor pressure (VP), dew point (DP), and relative humidity (RH).

the work in hand and the accuracy required.

The vapor pressure indicates the quantity of water vapor held in a given volume. For many purposes it is of particular advantage to know what quantity of water vapor is involved rather than its pressure. At a constant vapor pressure the relative humidity rises when the dry bulb temperature falls. This can be seen on Fig. 2–8 if the abscissa is followed to the left at a vapor pressure of, for example, 20 mbar. At a point between 17°C and 18°C DB, the relative humidity reaches 100 percent, which is saturation with water vapor; this is the dew point. If the DB now falls further, water condenses because the DB is below the dew point. The humidity may therefore be measured either by recording DB and WB temperatures or by estimating the dew point, because the latter is directly related to the vapor pressure and therefore gives a measure of the absolute humidity.

The difference between the saturation vapor pressure and the actual absolute vapor pressure is termed the "saturation deficit." This is sometimes referred to as a percentage, when it is equal to 100 percent minus the relative humidity, in percent. At 25°C, for example, the saturation vapor pressure is about 32 mbar. The previous example of 20 mbar water vapor pressure therefore represents at 25°C a saturation deficit of 32 − 20 = 12 mbar. This is a measure of the drying power available, because it indicates how much more water vapor can still be formed at the current temperature.

Other factors that influence evaporative heat transfer are also given in Table 2–1. The concept of "percent wetted area" is analogous to the area for the exchange of sensible heat. When sweating occurs at submaximal rates there is not a continuous film of sweat over the surface. However, an equivalent area of completely wetted surface can be estimated. Air movement is important in removing water vapor from its site of formation at the skin. It leads to an increase in the vapor pressure gradient, which is the driving force producing vaporization. The degree to which evaporative heat loss can occur varies considerably among different species. The evaporation takes place either on the animal's surface or in the upper respiratory tract.

Cutaneous Evaporative Loss

The rates of cutaneous water loss that are achieved under hot conditions are given for several animals in Fig. 2–9. One of the consequences of the range of potential evaporative losses in different species is that some animals can extend their control of body temperature into higher levels of environmental temperature that can produce hyperthermia in other animals. In spite of the lack of functional sweat glands in some species, all animals lose water through the

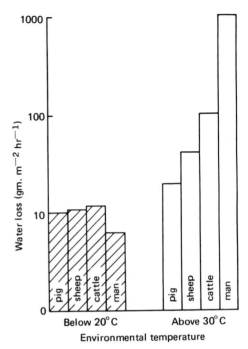

Fig. 2–9. Water loss (gm. m^{-2} hr^{-1}) through the skin in different species under cool (shaded bars) and hot conditions. Note the small effect of heat on the pig's evaporative loss compared to that of sheep, cattle, and man (logarithmic scale) (Mount, 1968b, *Adaptation of domestic animals*, E. S. E. Hafez, ed., Philadelphia: Lea and Febiger, p. 285).

skin by diffusion. Man has the capacity to sweat copiously from numerous eccrine glands distributed over the body surface, and he can survive in dry heat at 50°C or more with a normal deep body temperature. The pig, however, can lose only small amounts of water from the skin surface. The pig has eccrine sweat glands only on the snout, and some apocrine glands over the body surface. These apocrine glands produce very little secretion even under intense stimulation from drugs, and they do not appear to have a thermoregulatory function. When a pig is kept under hot dry conditions it readily becomes hyperthermic. The body temperature can be held within normal limits, however, if the animal is provided with some source of water, either wallows, sprays, mud, or urine, with which it can wet the body surface. Humid heat restricts evaporative loss more than dry heat because the higher environmental humidity reduces the difference of vapor pressure between the body surface and the environment and so reduces the rate of vaporization.

The actual site of vaporization is important in determining just how much of the evaporative heat is lost to the environment through this mode of heat transfer. Evaporation that takes place on the surface of bare skin, as in man, causes the heat of vaporization to be taken up from the body to a very large degree so that maximum cooling is achieved, although a small part of the heat is also taken up from the surrounding air. The precise site of vaporization makes a considerable difference to the cooling effect on an animal with a coat, however. For example, sweating in cattle, with evaporation at the skin surface, leads to considerable cooling of the body. The vaporization of rain water at the surface of a coat, in contrast, leads to heat being taken up from the coat and the surrounding air, with only minor effect on the skin tissues and peripheral blood circulation. The heat exchange of sheep is more complex because when the fleece becomes wet, heat is liberated from an exothermic reaction between water and wool, as a transient effect. This warming is superimposed on the cooling effect of evaporative heat loss.

Respiratory Evaporative Loss

Considerations similar to those discussed for the evaporation of sweat at the body surface also apply to evaporative heat transfer from the upper respiratory tract. The continuous respiratory movement of air over the surface of the respiratory tract produces a situation somewhat similar to that of forced convection enhancing evaporation at the skin surface. The subject has been discussed in some detail for man by Walker et al. (1961).

They are primarily concerned with the exchange and conservation of heat and water vapor in the airways.

The conditioning of inspired air is so efficient that even when the ambient air is at $-100°C$ it is heated to body temperature and becomes saturated with water vapor by the time it reaches the alveoli. During expiration, the air encounters the mucosa, which is cooled by inspiration. Some sensible heat now passes back to the mucosa, and some condensation of water takes place with the release of latent heat. The difference between the initial sensible and evaporative heat transfer to the inspired air and the transfer of some of this heat back to the mucosa during expiration is the respiratory heat loss. The net quantity of heat lost per unit volume respired is a function of the environmental temperature and humidity; the warmer and more humid the air, the smaller the net heat loss.

A number of investigations have shown that when man breathes quietly under equable conditions the temperature of the expired air falls from $37°C$ in the alveoli to about $32°C$ by the time it leaves the mouth or nose. At an ambient temperature of $-20°C$ to $-30°C$ the temperature of the expired air falls to $26°C$ (Sibbons, 1970). The inspired air is warmed and humidified in the upper respiratory tract as a result of turbulent convection, which causes a large part of the air to come into close contact with the mucosa. As the temperature of the inspired air rises, its ability to hold water vapor increases, an effect that is shown quantitatively in Figs. 2–8 and 2–10. Figure 2–10 shows the increase in water vapor content that saturated air can take up as its temperature is raised by $5°C$, and how much greater the increase is at higher as compared with lower temperatures. Conversely, greater condensation occurs from saturated air at the higher temperature when the temperature falls by a given amount.

This countercurrent exchange function is performed nearly as well during mouth breathing as during nasal breathing. Schmidt-

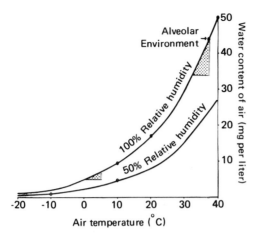

Fig. 2–10. Relation of water content of air to air temperature. A comparison of the height of the stippled triangles illustrates the difference in the amount of water condensed (cross lines) when the temperature of saturated air is lowered 5°C from body temperature (37°C) and 5°C from 5°C (Walker et al., 1961).

Nielsen et al. (1970) have investigated the respiratory countercurrent exchange of heat and water in birds and mammals with particular reference to the desert, where the conservation of water is so important for survival. They have found that the temperature of air expired by birds is closer to the environmental temperature than to the deep body temperature. Moreover, the air expired by small rodents is on occasion even cooler than the inspired air because of the evaporation of water from the nasal mucosa. In an environment at 15°C and 25 percent relative humidity, the amount of water recondensed during expiration is 74 percent of the water added to the air inspired by the cactus wren, and 83 percent is recovered by the kangaroo rat. Of the total sensible and evaporative heat added to the inspired air, 75 percent of the heat added on inspiration is recovered by the cactus wren during expiration, and 88 percent is recovered by the kangaroo rat. These amounts constitute a saving of 16 percent on the current metabolic heat production. A man breathing dry air at 0°C loses nearly one-fifth of his metabolic heat production through heating and humidification of the respiratory air. Even more would be lost if countercurrent heat exchange did not take place.

The sensible heat transfer involved in the warming of the respired air is relatively small when compared with the evaporative heat transfer. The heat capacity of air is approximately 1 J gm^{-1} °C^{-1}. Therefore, 500 ml of air (an average tidal volume for man, about 0.63 gm air at 200°C) requires only 10.7 J to warm it from 20°C to 37°C. At 15 respirations per minute, a heating rate of 2.7 W is needed to warm the inspired air to 37°C. If the air is expired at 32°C, five-seventeenths of this heat is retained because of countercurrent heat exchange, leaving approximately 2 W as the net requirement for warming respired air at an ambient temperature of 20°C. The evaporative transfer in respired air can be calculated assuming the ambient relative humidity to be 40–50 percent at a temperature of 20°C, with a corresponding vapor pressure of 11 mbar, and assuming the expired air to be saturated at 32°C, with a water vapor pressure of about 48 mbar. At a respiratory minute volume of 7.5 liters (that is, the volume of air respired in one minute), the water loss is about $7.5 \times (48 - 11/1000) = 0.28$ liter of vapor per minute, or 400 liters per day, equivalent to a mass of about 300 gm. A latent heat of vaporization of 2420 J gm^{-1} results in a rate of heat loss of 8.4 W, about four times the sensible heat loss under these conditions. Conditioning the inspired air at an ambient temperature of 20°C therefore requires about 11 W net, approximately 10 percent of the resting metabolism.

In a hot environment, the respiratory heat loss depends on the ambient humidity; at high humidities, evaporative heat loss is reduced. If air at a temperature exceeding body temperature and saturated with water vapor is inspired, there is a net gain of heat by the organism. At lower humidities, although the air temperature may be above body temperature, net evaporative loss occurs. At 42°C and 50 percent relative humidity, for example, there is a net evaporative loss that cools the mucosa to 35°C, and about 10 percent of the water evaporated from the mucosa on inspiration is recovered by the mucosa during expiration.

In some animals, an increased respiratory minute volume, which leads to greater respiratory heat loss, is an important adaptation to hot conditions. In the dog it takes the characteristic form of panting, which consists of shallow, rapid respiratory movements. The tidal air in panting is small, with the consequence that if the volume does not greatly exceed that of the respiratory dead space then excessive removal of carbon dioxide from the alveolar air does not occur. Excessive removal leads to respiratory alkalosis and disturbed acid–base balance. Similar rapid, shallow breathing also occurs in other animals, such as the sheep and pig, but the characteristic form of panting, with considerable evaporation from the protruding tongue and open mouth, is seen in its most highly developed form in the dog. The additional work involved in the rapid shallow panting of the dog is minimal. When cattle are exposed to high temperatures the respiratory rate at first increases, with little change in depth. As the animal's body temperature becomes progressively higher, however, the respiratory pattern changes to slower, deep respirations. It is at this stage that the acid–base balance becomes disturbed by respiratory alkalosis. Man pants only in extreme conditions; his capacity for cutaneous evaporative loss substantially exceeds in cooling power the evaporative loss associated with panting.

Calorimetry

"Calorimetry" is the term applied to the measurement of the exchange of heat. The various methods of calorimetry used in the past and those in current use have been adequately described in many textbooks and other publications; reference may be had to Lusk (1928), Brody (1945), Kleiber (1961), and Blaxter (1967). Attention is drawn to these methods here in order to indicate the range of approach to measuring heat production and heat loss in the whole animal. This is obviously of the greatest importance in assessing the effects of environment, nutrition, activity, and other factors on energy exchange. The choice of the method to be employed in any particular case depends on the sort of investigation in hand.

The types of calorimeter used for animals and man are either direct or indirect in their mode of operation. The direct calorimeter, as its name implies, measures heat exchange directly. It is the first type of calorimeter to have been employed, in the eighteenth century (Mount, 1968a). Indirect calorimetry involves the estimation of energy exchanges from the measurement of material exchanges.

There are two main types of direct calorimeter: one depends on absorbing the animal's heat loss and measuring it as a rise in temperature in the absorbing medium. The other depends on measuring the temperature difference produced across a layer surrounding the animal as the result of heat flow from the animal to its surroundings. The most celebrated instrument of the first kind has been the Atwater-Rosa-Benedict apparatus, in which heat is removed in circulating water (Atwater and Benedict, 1905; and see Lusk, 1928). Similar methods have been used by Armsby and Fries (1903) for cattle. Capstick (1921), Capstick and Wood (1922), and Deighton (1937) have made measurements on the pig in a calorimeter developed initially by Hill and Hill (1914). Also belonging to this class is the "air" calorimeter of Kelly et al. (1963), which is similar to that of Auguet and Lefèvre (1929). In this apparatus, the animal's heat loss is measured from the temperature rise in a ventilating air stream. Large "heat sink" calorimeters of the circulating water variety have been used recently for continuously measuring heat loss from pigs living in the apparatus for several weeks at a time (Mount, 1968a).

The other method of direct calorimetry was first used by Richet (1889) and Rubner (1894), who estimated the rate of heat flow from the temperature gradient across concentrically arranged air spaces around the calorimeter. Day and Hardy (1942) used the same principle for measuring heat loss from babies, and Prouty et al. (1949) made an animal calorimeter on similar lines. Their apparatus consisted of inner and outer copper cylinders, fixed in relation to each other. Heat flow from inside the inner cylinder produced a temperature difference across the layer of air between the two cylinders. In practice, therefore, the heat flow was determined as directly proportional to this temperature difference, which was measured by thermocouples. An electric fan blowing air on the outer cylinder maintained the outer shell at room temperature, and the shell and fan thus constituted a heat absorber of large capacity.

The concentric shell type of apparatus was succeeded by the accurate gradient layer calorimeter of Benzinger and Kitzinger (1949, 1963); Pullar (1958) also described a gradient layer calorimeter. Hammel and Hardy (1963) used a gradient layer calorimeter, coupled with oxygen and carbon dioxide measurement, to assess thermoregulatory responses in the dog. In these calorimeters, the temperature difference across a thin layer of material lining the inside of the chamber was measured by numerous thermocouples distributed over its whole area, so that the animal's heat loss could be accurately integrated.

Calorimeters of the direct variety can be calibrated from the dissipation of heat from electric heaters in which the energy liberated can be accurately measured. The evaporative component of heat loss can be assessed by varying the known rate of evaporation of water (Benzinger and Kitzinger, 1963; Mount, 1968a).

Distinct from these direct calorimetry approaches, which may be termed "heat sink" and "thermal gradient" methods, are the systems of indirect calorimetry. These again fall into two main groups: one is respiration calorimetry, and the other depends on the carbon and nitrogen analysis of food intake. The latter type may often be combined either with respiration calorimetry or with carcass analysis (Blaxter, 1967).

Respiration calorimetry in the form of measuring oxygen consumption is very widely used to determine heat production in either closed-circuit or open-circuit systems. Developed from the early apparatus of Reignault and Reiset (1849), the closed-circuit method, in which the animal is totally enclosed in a chamber forming part of the gas circuit, has led to the development and use of apparatuses of high accuracy (Brody, 1945; Alexander, 1961; Blaxter, 1967). Open-circuit systems have evolved from designs originally used by Haldane and by Pettenkofer (see Kleiber, 1961, p. 63).

The rate of oxygen consumption is commonly used as a measure of metabolism. When an animal is resting or moving so that no external work is done, the rate of heat production can be equated with the rate of oxygen consumption by using a value for the quantity of heat liberated when a unit quantity of oxygen is consumed. If the animal is doing external work, however, for example, climbing a slope or working a machine, the whole of its metabolic rate does not appear as heat. The metabolic rate then equals the heat produced in the animal plus the external work done. The calorific value of oxygen varies with the particular combination of foodstuffs being metabolized. It is higher when these are largely fat, with a range from 21.1 to 19.7 kJ/liter. The combination actually involved can be determined from the nonprotein respiratory quotient, which requires the measurement of carbon dioxide production simultaneously with that of oxygen consumption (Lusk, 1928).

The measurement of carbon dioxide production by itself is not altogether satisfactory as a measure of metabolism unless much greater care is taken than with oxygen consumption, particularly with respect to the length of the measurement period and the stability of conditions. This is because the organism contains large quantities of carbon dioxide that are either free in the body fluids or bound as bicarbonate. Variations between the quantities held in these capacities interfere with the determination of the rate at which carbon dioxide is being produced from metabolic processes. Animals cannot store corresponding amounts of oxygen, so a similar difficulty does not arise when metabolic rate is determined from oxygen consumption.

Indirect calorimeters are usually calibrated by the alcohol check, which is fully described by Hammel and Hardy (1963). From the weights of alcohol burnt in a lamp in the calorimeter, the quantities of oxygen consumed and carbon dioxide produced can be calculated. These can then be compared with the quantities measured by the calorimeter. The alcohol lamp may also be used for calibrating a direct calorimeter, using the known value of 20.4 kJ liberated for each liter of oxygen burning alcohol.

Partitional Calorimetry

In an extensive series of papers, Winslow, Herrington, and Gagge developed the basis of partitional calorimetry in its application to man (see Mount, 1968a, for references). Their method was basically to expose the subject to an environment in which the components responsible for heat exchange by convection and radiation could be varied independently of each other. They were then able to write heat balance equations for different sets of conditions, and so to arrive at the heat exchange taking place through each of the channels of convection, radiation, and

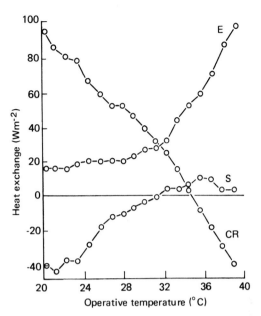

Fig. 2–11. The thermal exchanges of nude human subjects at various operative temperatures. E, heat transfer by evaporation; S, storage heat (body cooling or warming); CR, heat transfer by radiation and convection (Gagge et al., 1938, *Am. J. Physiol.* **124**: 30).

evaporation (conduction played only a small part in their experiments). The system they used consisted of an enclosure lined by polished copper plates that reflected heat from external radiant heaters on to the subject. The reflected heat then largely determined the subject's radiant environment. The mean radiant temperature was integrated by a hemispherical, convex, reflecting surface mounted above the enclosure. This and the subject's mean skin temperature and effective radiating area were taken as the quantities governing radiant heat exchange. Convective heat exchange depended on air temperature and the air movement rate in the vicinity of the subject. Figure 2–11 illustrates the partition of heat loss from man under these conditions over a range of operative temperatures.

CHAPTER 3

Metabolic Rate, Thermal Insulation, and the
Assessment of Environment

Metabolic Rate and Heat Loss
at High Temperatures

"Hot" is a relative term in environmental physiology, just as it is in physics. For the newborn pig or newborn baby an environmental temperature of 32°C coupled with low air movement appears to be a "comfortable" environment, but for the mature pig or man it is "hot." A further distinction is that under dry conditions the taxing effects of a given high temperature are greater for the pig than for man because the pig cannot sweat. "High temperature" should therefore be considered with reference not to actual temperatures but rather to particular zones of temperature. For the animal under discussion, these zones have been described in terms of thermal neutrality, least thermoregulatory effort, or comfort. These zones occur at different places on the temperature scale not only for different species but also for animals of the same species that are at

different stages of development or adaptation. There has been some preliminary discussion of this subject in Chapter 1.

Thermal Neutrality

The concept of thermal neutrality has arisen from the changes that occur in a homeotherm's metabolic rate when its environmental temperature is varied. At low temperatures, the animal's metabolic rate is elevated in response to thermoregulatory demand: body temperature is maintained at the expense of increased heat production. The degree of cold the animal can tolerate is determined by its maximum rate of cold-stimulated heat production and by its thermal insulation. Figure 3–1 illustrates this point for the newborn pig, which is particularly sensitive to cold. It also shows that as the temperature rises the "thermal demand of the environment" decreases; that is, less

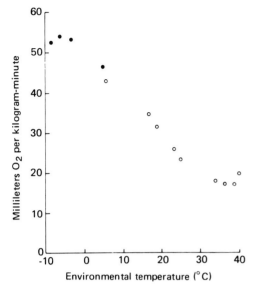

Fig. 3–1. Maximum and minimum metabolic rates in the newborn pig, 2 days old and weighing about 1.7 kg. One pig (●) was exposed to a decreasing environmental temperature to detect the maximum metabolic rate, and the other pig (○) was exposed to a rising temperature to detect the minimum rate (Mount and Stephens, 1970, *J. Physiol.* (*London* **207:** 417).

heat production is required for the maintenance of body temperature and the metabolic rate falls. A point is then reached at which the metabolic rate is minimum. The actual level of the minimum depends on a number of factors, particularly the level of feeding. If the level of feeding is high, the minimal metabolism is also high, an effect shown in Fig. 3–2. Both Figs. 3–1 and 3–2 also indicate that as the environmental temperature rises further, the metabolic rate first remains constant at its minimum value and then begins to increase. This increase is related to a rise in body temperature; that is, the animal is hyperthermic.

The zone of thermal neutrality, as originally defined, is that range of environmental temperature over which the metabolic rate is (1) constant, (2) at a minimum, and (3) independent of temperature. The width of such a zone varies considerably among different animals. It is very narrow in the

case of the pig and the mouse, for example, for these animals have little capacity for evaporative heat loss and consequently cannot dissipate heat readily under hot conditions. As the environmental temperature rises, therefore, they become hyperthermic after a much smaller temperature interval of neutrality than, for example, man. Man has considerable ability to sweat and so to dissipate heat. He thereby avoids hyperthermia until a much wider temperature span of neutrality has been crossed. A man at a high temperature may still be metabolizing at the minimal rate but may be avoiding the hyperthermic rise by sweating more than usual.

A zone with an upper limit set by the onset of increased evaporative loss is more likely to be neutral both in respect of human comfort and of animal productivity. As the result of a recent discussion (Mount, 1974), it has been concluded that it may be useful to define a number of environmental zones that are "neutral" in different respects. These

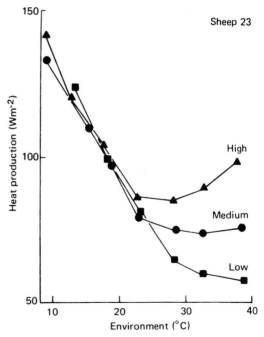

Fig. 3–2. The heat production of a sheep per square meter body surface at three feeding levels in relation to environmental temperature (Graham et al., 1959, *J. Agric. Sci., Camb.* **52:** 13).

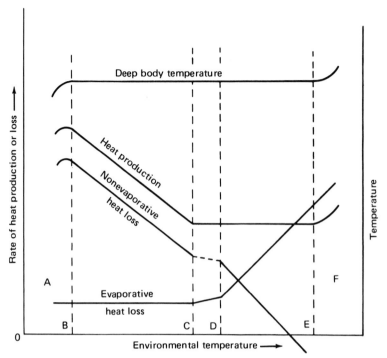

Fig. 3–3. Diagrammatic representation of relations between heat production, evaporative and nonevaporative heat loss, and deep body temperature in a homeothermic animal. (A) Zone of hypothermia; (B) temperature of summit metabolism and incipient hypothermia; (C) critical temperature; (D) temperature of marked increase in evaporative loss; (E) temperature of incipient hyperthermic rise; (F) zone of hyperthermia; (CD) zone of least thermoregulatory effort and minimal material demand; (CE) zone of minimal metabolism; (BE) thermoregulatory range (Mount, 1974).

are illustrated in Fig. 3–3, in which heat production and heat loss are related to environmental temperature:

1. Minimal metabolism; CE in Fig. 3–3
2. Least thermoregulatory effort, coinciding with minimal material demand either for food to meet cold demand or for water to meet high temperature demand; CD in Fig. 3–3
3. Zones defined for comfort, animal productivity, or other purposes not necessarily coinciding with either (1) or (2) above

Critical Temperature

The lower end of the zone of minimal metabolism is termed the "critical temperature." At temperatures below this level the animal's heat production must rise if body temperature is to be maintained. The critical temperature is also usually accepted as the point at which vasoconstriction occurs when the environmental temperature falls, and most experimental evidence endorses this view. This is not always the case, however. In experiments in which thin and fat men have been suspended in a water bath at different temperatures, it has been found that bath temperatures for maximum tissue insulation (vasoconstriction) and for the metabolic critical temperature are the same only for the thin men. The fat men increase their metabolic rates in water below 33°C but do not reach maximum tissue insulation until the water temperature is much lower than 33°C (Cannon and Keatinge, 1966).

The significance of vasodilatation above

the critical temperature is that the transfer of heat from the animal's core to the surface is facilitated by increased blood flow, with the result that the thermal conductance rises to a maximum value and heat loss through the sensible channels is increased. By this means, and as the result of a more extended posture that increases the surface area for heat exchange, the animal's deep body temperature remain steady as the environmental temperature continues to rise, although the rate of heat production remains constant at its maximum. The skin temperature rises and so maintains both the temperature difference with the environment and the sensible heat loss corresponding to that difference, in spite of the increase in environmental temperature (see Fig. 2–7). A further rise in environmental temperature leads to inadequate dissipation of heat in spite of the vasomotor and postural changes. The animal's deep body temperature then rises unless increased evaporative cooling takes place from respiratory or cutaneous surfaces.

A particular point arises with reference to the plot of sensible heat loss in Fig. 3–3. Figure 2–7 shows sensible heat loss from a pig; extrapolation of the straight line derived from points corresponding to the lower environmental temperatures, at which the animal is vasoconstricted, produces in that diagram an intercept on the temperature axis at the level of the deep body temperature. This is to be expected when only sensible heat loss is involved, as for example from a heated sphere, because when the environmental temperature reaches the required temperature of the sphere the heat input necessary to maintain that temperature is zero. The points corresponding to the higher temperature in Fig. 2–7 occur when the pig is vasodilated, and, because the animal's zone of minimal metabolism is narrow, this is also where the deep body temperature begins to rise. In Fig. 3–3, however, a rather wider zone of minimal metabolism (CE) is assumed for the purposes of the general case, and the sensible (nonevaporative) heat loss is shown remaining nearly constant from the

critical temperature (C) upward along the temperature scale for a short interval before resuming a decline. This interval corresponds to the onset of peripheral vasodilatation, which is probably accompanied by a small increase in evaporative loss. If vasodilatation should occur completely and at once at the critical temperature, the sensible loss line must rise sharply at that point and then decline again as the environmental temperature rises further. The probability is, however, that vasodilatation occurs over a finite temperature interval, as shown by the interrupted line in Fig. 3–3.

Reference to Fig. 3–2 shows that as a consequence of a higher level of minimal metabolism at a higher level of feeding, the critical temperature is lower. For an animal fed at a higher level, therefore, the zone of minimal metabolism moves down the scale of environmental temperature; a temperature representing somewhat cool conditions for an animal on a low plane of nutrition constitutes a neutral or even a warm environment for the animal that is receiving more feed. Below the critical temperature, the animal's rate of heat loss is a function of the environment, and the thermal insulation can be calculated from the relation between heat loss and environmental temperature.

Thermal Conductance and Insulation

Whichever way the line relating sensible heat loss to environmental temperature changes at the critical temperature, when it begins to decline again with a further rise in temperature it does so along a steeper path. Provided the animal is still within the zone of minimal metabolism, so that it is not hyperthermic, the intercept on the temperature axis is at the same point because the deep body temperature has not changed. The slopes of the line below and above the criti-

cal temperature give the thermal conductance in each situation in respect of sensible
heat flow (H_N):

$$C = \frac{H_N}{T_B - T_E} \qquad (3\text{–}1)$$

where C = thermal conductance
T_B = deep body temperature
T_E = environmental temperature

A difficulty arises here. The thermal
conductance is equivalent to an overall heat
transfer coefficient for the animal and has the
dimensions of heat flow per unit temperature
difference. However, although heat transfer
from the core to the cutaneous and respiratory surfaces is all in the sensible mode, the
heat that flows from those surfaces to the
environment is in both sensible and evaporative modes. The sensible and evaporative
heat transfers are in parallel and are therefore additive, and their magnitudes may be
calculated from sensible and evaporative
transfer coefficients. These coefficients, however, have different dimensions, because the
sensible coefficient involves temperature and
the evaporative coefficient involves vapor
pressure. The reciprocals of the coefficients
give the resistances to transfer, and these are
referred to as the "sensible insulation" and
the "evaporative resistance."

Sensible Insulation

The total sensible insulation (R) from
the animal's core to the environment can be
divided into two additive insulations in series, the internal (R_I) and the external (R_E):

$$R = R_I + R_E \qquad (3\text{–}2)$$

R_I then involves H, the total heat flow,
but R_E involves only the sensible component
of heat loss from the animal's surfaces.
When the mean skin temperature is represented as T_S:

$$R_I = \frac{T_B - T_S}{H} = \frac{T_B - T_S}{H_N + H_E} \qquad (3\text{–}3)$$

and

$$R_E = \frac{T_S - T_E}{H_N} \qquad (3\text{–}4)$$

where H_E is the evaporative heat transfer.

The internal insulation, R_I, lies between the animal's core and the body surface. In this context, the core means heat-
producing tissues. The distribution of the
core therefore varies depending on muscular
activity. When the organism is resting, the
brain and thoracic and abdominal viscera are
the chief centers of heat production. During
activity, however, heat is also produced in
the muscles. In both cases subcutaneous fat
and other tissues provide internal insulation,
with circulating blood as the principal channel of heat transfer to the surface. Peripheral
vasoconstriction leads to reduced blood flow
through the skin and superficial tissues, so
that subcutaneous fat is effective as insulation. Cooling of the body "shell," as opposed to the core (see Fig. 2–1), leads to
further reduction in heat loss. When peripheral vasodilatation occurs under conditions
of warmth or activity, however, the blood
flow through the fat layer to the surface
effectively "short circuits" the insulation of
the fat layer and the rise in skin temperature
leads to a rise in heat loss.

When the skin temperature rises, the
ensuing increased heat loss leads in turn to
cooling. The resultant level of skin temperature depends on the rate of heat loss and
the rate at which warm blood from the core
reaches the skin. The rate of heat loss depends on sweating and evaporation as well
as on sensible transfer by radiation and convection. A vigorously exercising man under
cool conditions may have a low skin temperature in spite of vasodilatation, whereas
a resting man under hot conditions, also
vasodilated, has a high skin temperature.

The external insulation, R_E, includes
the insulation offered by coat or clothing

(R_C), which is basically trapped still air, plus the insulation from the exposed surfaces to the surroundings (R_A), and as these are in series:

$$R_E = R_C + R_A \qquad (3\text{--}5)$$

A temperature gradient exists through R_C, from the skin surface to the surface of the coat or clothing, and only the sensible component of heat transfer is involved in the production of this gradient:

$$R_C = \frac{T_S - T_C}{H_N}$$

where T_C is the surface temperature of the coat or clothing.

R_A is sometimes referred to as "air insulation" or "ambient insulation" (Blaxter, 1967; Hey et al., 1970). Because it includes convective and radiative parts it is perhaps most appropriately referred to as the "air–ambient insulation." The convective component of R_A depends on the boundary layer of air around the body or organism. The boundary layer is a layer of air, several millimeters thick on average, that offers convective insulation because it is stable in a direction normal to the surface. Direct visualization by Schlieren photography has shown that the layer is not stationary in a direction parallel to the surface, but that it streams over the surface in consequence of natural convection caused by warming by the organism (Lewis et al., 1969). This does not prevent the layer from acting as thermal insulation in a direction normal to the surface. The thickness of the boundary layer depends on the roughness, shape, and size of the surface and is approximately proportional to the square root of the diameter. A lower radius of curvature is therefore associated with higher convective heat loss.

The radiative component of the air–ambient insulation per unit area can be derived from a simple form of the equation for radiant exchange given earlier (p. 13):

$$H_R = \sigma F(T_S^4 - T_E^4) \qquad (3\text{--}6)$$

In this case both the air and mean radiant temperatures are assumed to be equal and to give an environmental temperature T_E. To a close approximation, the difference between the fourth powers of the skin and environmental temperatures is proportional to the difference between the temperatures, for small differences. Burton and Edholm (1955) have shown that when $(T_S - T_E)$ is used instead of $(T_S^4 - T_E^4)$ the departure from linearity is less than 5 percent when values of $(T_S - T_E)$ of 10°C and 20°C are compared. The equation can then be written:

$$\sigma(T_S^4 - T_E^4) = 4\sigma T^3(T_S - T_E) \qquad (3\text{--}7)$$

where $T = (T_S + T_E)/2$

The quantity $4\sigma T^3$ gives the radiant exchange for each 1°C difference between skin and environmental temperatures; when $T = 27$°C this is 6.0 W m^{-2} °C^{-1}.

Equation (3–6) may therefore be written:

$$H_R = kF(T_S - T_E) \qquad (3\text{--}8)$$

where k is a constant of proportionality involving the Stefan-Boltzmann constant. The radiative insulation, R_R, is then given by the relation analogous to Ohm's Law (see p. 9):

$$R_R = \frac{T_S - T_E}{H_R} = \frac{1}{kF} \qquad (3\text{--}9)$$

showing that it depends on the emissivities of the animal and environmental surfaces. R_R is the highest when the emissivities (and therefore the absorptivities) are low, because then there is minimum radiant heat transfer for a given temperature difference. The combined air–ambient insulation at low air movement and in a chamber with "black" walls, that is, walls of high emissivity, has been calculated as 0.12°C m^2 W^{-1} for man (Winslow et al., 1940), and similar values have been calculated for calves, steers, and pigs. From measurements made on sheep in chambers with partly polished walls, and therefore with lower emissivity, the air–ambient insulation has a higher value, as expected, at 0.14 to 0.16 °C m² W⁻¹ (Joyce et al., 1966).

The conductive component of the external insulation takes the place of the air–ambient insulation in those areas of the animal in direct contact with solid surfaces. Because the animal's surface and the solid surface both tend toward the same temperature, the conductive insulation is most appropriately indicated by the ratio of the temperature gradient to the heat flow through the floor. This quantity equals the thermal insulation of the material of the floor. The thermal capacity of the floor must also be taken into account because this acts as a heat sink (or source) until temperature equilibrium is reached. In many instances, the conductive insulation per unit area often approximates to the air–ambient insulation per unit area, although on such insulated surfaces as bedding it is considerably greater. In practice it is best determined empirically, in a particular situation, because it involves the multidirectional heat flows characteristic of volume conductivity, which make theoretical treatment difficult. Haartsen (1967) has measured the rates of heat loss to piggery floors from a bag of water maintained thermostatically at a given temperature. His results show both the initial floor warming of the heat capacity effect and the eventual equilibrium rates of heat loss that depend on the floor insulation.

From Eqs. (3–2), (3–3), and (3–4), the sum of the internal and external sensible insulations gives the total sensible insulation:

$$R = \left(\frac{T_B - T_S}{H_N + H_E}\right) + \left(\frac{T_S - T_E}{H_N}\right) \qquad (3\text{–}10)$$

As pointed out by Hey et al. (1970), this becomes:

$$R = \frac{(T_B - T_E) - H_E \cdot R_I}{H_N} \qquad (3\text{–}11)$$

because the denominators (the internal and external sensible heat flows) in Eq. (3–10)

differ from each other. The term $H_E \cdot R_I$ appears because the evaporation of water from the skin accounts for some of the heat passing from the core to the skin. $H_E \cdot R_I$ has the dimensions of temperature (°C). It equals the amount by which the core–environment temperature difference must be diminished to give the difference corresponding to the passage through the core–environment insulation of only that part of the total heat flow lost from the animal's surface as sensible heat. $H_E \cdot R_I$ becomes important under hot conditions when the core and environmental temperatures are close together and particularly noticeable when $T_E = T_S$ and H_N is zero. There is then still a gradient between core and skin temperature (unless R_I is negligible) caused by evaporative heat loss from the skin. Equation (3–11) shows that H_N is zero when T_E is somewhat less than T_B, the exact difference being given by $H_E \cdot R_I$. The results in Fig. 3–4 are in accordance with this conclusion. In this diagram sensible heat loss from babies is related to $(T_B - T_E)$, and the intercept of the plot on the temperature axis is above $(T_B - T_E) = 0$. Therefore, T_E is less than T_B at the intercept. This rather precise consideration qualifies the statements made earlier to the effect that for sensible heat loss the intercept is at the deep body temperature, which is the case only if there is no evaporative loss, as in the heated sphere. Even in a nonsweating animal, such as the pig, however, there is a small cutaneous water loss as well as respiratory evaporative loss. Therefore, the correct statement is that the intercept is close to but just below deep body temperature, by an amount equal to $H_E \cdot R_I$.

The sensible (nonevaporative) heat loss line in Fig. 3–3 refers to heat loss from the animal's surface to the environment, that is, to H_N; however at equilibrium at any one temperature the metabolic heat production equals H, the total heat loss. The H_N line has an intercept close to the deep body temperature on the temperature axis because it is assumed that when the environmental temperature reaches that point, temperatures a hypothetical situation, because it applies strictly only when there is no evaporative heat loss. In the real situation in an animal with evaporative heat loss, Eq. (3–11) shows that the intercept is the deep body temperature only when the internal insulation R_I is zero. This condition is approached when there is a very large skin blood flow.

This concept is used in deriving the thermal circulation index, TCI:

$$TCI = \frac{\text{external insulation}}{\text{internal insulation}}$$

$$= \frac{(T_S - T_E)/H_N}{(T_B - T_S)/H}$$

In practice, to the extent that H_N approximates to H, as in the pig where cutaneous evaporation is small, the expression becomes:

$$TCI \simeq \frac{T_S - T_E}{T_B - T_S} \qquad (3\text{--}12)$$

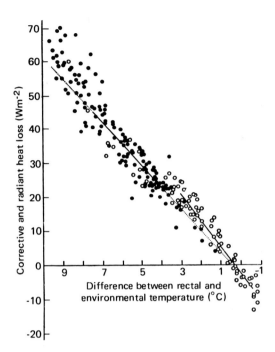

which has been termed the "uncorrected thermal circulation index" (Hey and Katz 1970). Figure 3–5 gives skin temperature against environmental temperature and the thermal circulation index for the young pig. Above 33°C the index shows a marked upward turn toward infinity (when $T_B = T_S$). This marks the vasodilatation and increased internal thermal conductance that indicate the critical temperature. Evidence from the determination of metabolic rate in the young pig indicates a critical temperature of about 34°C (Mount, 1968a) so that information from both temperature and metabolism give similar results in this particular case. The usefulness of the TCI is that an estimate of metabolic rate is not required. It is valid, however, only under equilibrium conditions and not during fluctuations of temperature.

Fig. 3–4. The relation between the net temperature gradient and total heat loss by convection and radiation in 12 babies 0–14 days old and weighing between 1.8 and 2.2 kg. Results obtained when rectal temperature (T_r) is 37.2°C or more are indicated by open symbols. The lower line is the best-fit relation for all the data obtained when T_r is less than 37.2°C (mean 36.9°C) and the operative environmental temperature (T_e) is between 29.5°C and 33°C. The relation has a slope that is equivalent to an insulation of 0.164°C m² W⁻¹ and an intercept on the x axis of 0.26°C. The results obtained when T_e is below 29.5°C nearly all lie above the dotted extension of this line. Most of the babies were physically active in an environment as cool as this. The upper line is the best-fit relation for all the data obtained when T_r is 37.2°C or more (mean 37.4°C) and T_e is between 34°C and 37.5°C. This relation has a slope that is equivalent to an insulation of 0.130°C m² W⁻¹ and an intercept of 0.22°C on the x axis. This intercept differs significantly from zero ($P < 0.05$). The air speed was 4–5 cm sec⁻¹ (Hey et al., 1970).

Evaporative Heat Loss

are equal throughout the body. Therefore, skin temperature is uniform and equal to the deep body temperature. This is largely

When the sensible heat loss declines as the environmental temperature rises above

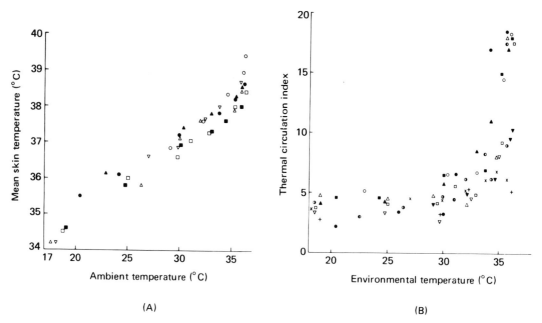

Fig. 3–5. (A) Skin temperature (mean value from head, both flanks, back, and abdomen) of 12 pigs up to 9 days old plotted against environmental temperature. Each symbol refers to a different pig. (B) The relation between the thermal circulation index and environmental temperature for the 12 newborn pigs referred to in 3–5(A) (Mount, 1964b, *J. Physiol. (London)* **170:** 286, by permission).

the level at which vasodilatation occurs, the deep body temperature remains stable. The metabolic rate, however, continues at the constant minimum level characteristic of thermal neutrality because evaporative heat loss increases. The sum of sensible and evaporative losses equals the rate of heat production, as shown in Fig. 3–3, provided that the mean body temperature remains constant so that heat storage does not occur. When the environmental temperature rises above the body temperature so that there is a sensible heat transfer from the environment, body temperature can still be maintained constant in a strongly sweating species, such as man, although a sensible heat load from the environment as well as the metabolic heat must be dissipated through the evaporative channel. The effectiveness of evaporative heat transfer depends on an adequate vapor pressure difference between the animal's respiratory and cutaneous surfaces, on the one hand, and the environment, on the other.

As the temperature of the surroundings rises still further, the limit of evaporative heat loss is reached. Body temperature then begins to rise, accompanied by the hyperthermic rise in metabolic rate, which leads to a positive feedback between mutually accelerating metabolic rate and hyperthermia. This situation is reached at a lower temperature in an animal with limited evaporative heat loss, such as the pig. Hyperthermia may then ensue before environmental temperature reaches body temperature.

Evaporative Resistance

The resistance offered to the transfer of heat by the vaporization of water on a surface can be formulated in a manner analogous to that for sensible insulation. Instead of the temperature difference that operates in sensible insulation [see Eq. (3–3)], there is a difference of water vapor pressure, and instead of the diffusion of heat there is the diffusion of water vapor. The evaporative resistance, R_V, is then given by:

$$R_V = \frac{P_S - P_A}{E} \qquad (3\text{–}13)$$

where P_S = mean vapor pressure at skin

P_A = mean environmental vapor pressure

E = rate of diffusion of water vapor

The value of E increases as air movement increases and decreases when coat or clothing are interposed between the skin and the surrounding air, with corresponding inverse effects on the evaporative resistance R_V.

The value of P_S, the mean vapor pressure at the skin surface, has been discussed by Burton and Edholm (1955). They point out that the skin surface can be considered as a mosaic of small completely wetted areas separated by completely dry areas. The vapor pressure over the wetted areas is then assumed to be the saturated vapor pressure at skin temperature, and the vapor pressure over the dry areas to be that of the environment. This is clearly an oversimplification. It does not take into account the diffusion of water through the skin, which takes place over all areas, including the postulated dry areas. However, the concept allows an approximate calculation that has the merit of usefulness. The effective wetted area of a man who is not sweating falls to a minimum of about 10 percent of the maximum that is reached when the body is completely covered by nonevaporated sweat. The diffusing water vapor spreads out laterally from the wetted areas, and at a short distance from the skin a uniform mean vapor pressure is reached. On the basis of proportions this pressure has the value:

$$P_S = \frac{W \cdot P_{\text{sat}S} + (100 - W)P_A}{100} \qquad (3\text{–}14)$$

where W = wetted areas as a percentage of the total

$P_{\text{sat}S}$ = saturated vapor pressure at skin temperature over the wetted areas

When the wetted area is small, the environmental vapor pressure, P_A, has a marked effect on the mean vapor pressure at the skin. It should be noted that the absolute vapor pressures, and not relative humidities, are used in this calculation because the relative humidity gives only the percentage of the saturation vapor pressure at a given temperature.

The vapor pressure gradient that provides the driving force in evaporation is given from Eq. (3–14) by:

$$(P_S - P_A) = \frac{W \cdot P_{\text{sat}S} + (100 - W)P_A}{100} - P_A$$

$$= \frac{W(P_{\text{sat}S} - P_A)}{100} \qquad (3\text{–}15)$$

Equation (3–13), which gives the evaporative resistance, then becomes:

$$R_V = \frac{W(P_{\text{sat}S} - P_A)}{100 \cdot E} \qquad (3\text{–}16)$$

The situation with respect to respiratory evaporative resistance corresponds to that for cutaneous evaporation. For evaporation from the respiratory tract (Burton and Edholm, 1955):

$$E = V(Q_{\text{sat}} - Q_A)K \qquad (3\text{–}17)$$

where V = respiratory ventilation per unit time

Q_{sat} = quantity of water vapor in the saturated expired air

Q_A = quantity of water vapor in ambient air

K = evaporative heat transfer per unit mass of water evaporated

The respiratory evaporative resistance (R_{VR}) then takes the form:

$$R_{VR} = \frac{P_{\text{sat}R} - P_A}{V(Q_{\text{sat}} - Q_A)K} \qquad (3\text{–}18)$$

where $P_{\text{sat}R}$ = saturated vapor pressure in the expired air

with the result that R_{VR} decreases as the ventilation volume increases.

The evaporative resistance is formed by two resistances in series, the evaporative resistance of coat or clothing, R_{VC}, and the evaporative resistance of the air, R_{VA}. Air movement and other factors, such as size and shape, that affect the insulation of the boundary layer to convective heat transfer also have proportionally similar effects on the evaporative transfer. Although evaporative and sensible heat transfers may be described in different units, therefore, they nonetheless show similar degrees of variation when the organism is exposed to environmental changes that affect the boundary layer. The theoretical basis of the relation between the coefficients of convective and evaporative heat losses has been discussed by Rapp (1970). Coefficients of evaporative heat transfer have been discussed by Sibbons (1970).

Monteith (1973) has shown how a unified approach can be made to the resistances to the transfers of heat, mass (water vapor and CO_2), and momentum. Resistance to transfer is given by the diffusion path length divided by the diffusion coefficient, giving a quantity with the dimensions of (time) $\times$ (length)$^{-1}$, which is the reciprocal of velocity. This is the common measure of resistance and can be used not only in cases limited to molecular diffusion but also in any system where fluxes are uniquely related to gradients.

With the usual units, sensible insulation is expressed in °C m^2 W^{-1}. This can be put in terms of the common measure of resistance by multiplying by the volumetric heat capacity of air (density $\times$ specific heat at constant pressure). The value obtained is then directly comparable with that for evaporative resistance similarly expressed. It is necessary to choose an arbitrary value of ρC_p for air, for example, 1.21 kJ m^{-3} °C^{-1}, which is the value at 20°C. A unit of resistance $r = 1$ second cm^{-1} is then equivalent to an insulation $r/\rho C_p = 0.083$ °C m^2 W^{-1}. Using the resistance approach, Monteith also shows that the diffusion resistance for evaporation in even rapid respiration exceeds the boundary layer resistance of the skin by an order of magnitude. Therefore, when the skin is covered with sweat the res-

piratory evaporative loss is much smaller than the cutaneous evaporation rate.

The Assessment of Thermal Environment

There have been many attempts to formulate a unitary physiological temperature scale for the purpose of referring to the thermal characteristics of a given environment as a single quantity in relation to a living organism. The demand made by the environment on an animal to produce or to dissipate heat, and so to regulate its body temperature, is formed by the effects of all the factors that influence heat exchange through the several channels discussed above. It is tempting to think of a simple model that can integrate these components of the environment into an equivalent still-air temperature as an indicator of environmental thermal demand.

Equivalence between environments established in this way, however, as between a high-radiant–low-convective temperature combination, and a low-radiant–high-convective combination, applies only to the particular model used, owing to the laws governing heat transfer by radiation and convection. For example, a small sphere is more sensitive to a given change in convective environment than is a large sphere. Coefficients may be determined to relate the results obtained with the smaller sphere to the effect on the larger sphere, but to attempt such transformations in the case of animals of differing size, thermal insulation, and posture leads to considerable complications and gross inaccuracies. The alternative approach is to abandon the search for a unitary estimate of thermal demand. Instead, heat transfer should be estimated through each of the four channels of radiation, convection, conduction, and evaporation separately, and then a physiological assessment of the effects on the organism can be made (Mount, 1968a).

For man, however, Burton and Edholm (1955) describe a method of determining an "equivalent still-air temperature." This is derived by adding to air temperature, algebraically, a thermal-wind-decrement in temperature that allows for the effect of air movement. If an increment of temperature is now added to allow for radiation from the sun or elsewhere, the "equivalent still–shade temperature" is estimated. These formulations have considerable convenience in assessing man's insulation requirements in different environments.

An "effective temperature scale" has been developed as a sensory scale of warmth combining air temperature, air movement, and humidity into a single index (Chapter 10). The numerical value of the scale is the temperature of still air saturated with water vapor that induces a sensation of warmth or cold equal to that of the given condition. A "corrected effective temperature" that makes allowances for radiant heat has also been introduced (Bedford, 1946).

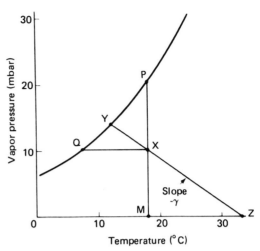

Fig. 3–6. The relationship between dry bulb temperature, wet bulb temperature, equivalent temperature, vapor pressure, and dew point. The point X represents air at 18°C and 10 mbar vapor pressure. The line YXZ with a slope of —γ gives the wet bulb temperature from Y (12°C) and the equivalent temperature from Z (33.3°C). The line QX gives the dew point temperature from Q (7.1°C). The line XO gives the saturation vapor pressure from P (20.6 mbar) (Monteith, 1973).

Apparent Equivalent Temperature

The term "equivalent temperature" has a special meaning in meteorological thermodynamics (Monteith, 1973; 1974). In Fig. 3–6, which corresponds with Fig. 2–8, the curve QYP gives the relation between saturation vapor pressure and DB temperature. X represents a sample of air at a DB temperature of M and a WB temperature of Y. If the state of the sample of air changes from X toward Y adiabatically (i.e., with the total heat content of the system remaining constant), it becomes cooler and its vapor pressure increases. Moving in the other direction, along the line YX from Y, water is condensed and the DB temperature rises until the produced line reaches zero vapor pressure at Z. At this point all the water vapor is condensed, and the temperature θ given by the point Z is called the "equivalent tem-

perature." The slope of the line YZ can be shown to be —γ, where γ is the psychrometer constant with a value of 0.66 mbar °C^{-1} at a 20°C temperature and a 1013 mbar pressure. The psychrometer constant multiplied by the difference between dry and wet bulb readings gives the difference between the saturation vapor pressure at the WB temperature and the actual vapor pressure of the sample of air. The equation of the line ZX can be written:

$$\theta = T + e/\gamma$$

where T = DB temperature
e = water vapor pressure

A numerical example can be given as follows: X represents air at 18°C and 10 mbar vapor pressure; the WB temperature Y is 12°C, and the equivalent temperature Z is 33.3°C. Q is the dew point temperature, 7.1°C, and P is the saturation vapor pressure of 20.6 mbar, with XM/PM giving the relative humidity. The equivalent temperature $\theta = 33.3°C$ indicates the enthalpy potential of the air sample, just as $T = 18°C$ represents the sensible heat transfer potential. The value of θ is that it provides a quantity to describe the heat balance of any surface from which water is evaporating, with adjustment for the diffusion resistances (see p. 34) of heat and vapor for the particular physical conditions. Monteith has thus achieved in principle the formulation of a unitary temperature scale, although some difficulties of measurement remain.

Operative Temperature

As opposed to the sensory effective temperature scale, the operative temperature scale (Gagge, 1940) provides a physical measure of the thermal environment. Operative temperature combines as a single variable the temperature equivalents of the radiant and the convective environments. This is achieved by using coefficients to relate radiant and convective heat exchanges to the differences between skin temperature, on the one side, and mean radiant and air temperatures, on the other. Although it is the difference between the fourth powers of the absolute temperatures that determines the radiant exchange, when the temperature differences are small the simple temperature difference itself can be used with only a small error, as discussed on p. 00 (Burton and Edholm, 1955).

$$T_0 = \frac{K_R T_W + K_C T_A}{K_R + K_C} \qquad (3\text{-}19)$$

where T_0 = operative temperature

K_R = coefficient of heat transfer by radiation

K_C = coefficient of heat transfer by convection for a given air movement rate

T_W = mean radiant temperature

T_A = air temperature

The following expression gives the operative temperature for man in terms of T_W, T_A, and V, the velocity of air movement:

$$T_0 = \frac{K_R}{K_0} T_W + \frac{K_C}{K_0}[(\sqrt{V/V_0})T_A -$$
$$[\sqrt{(V/V_0)} - 1]T_S] \quad (3\text{-}20)$$

where $K_0 = K_R + k_C \sqrt{V_0}$

$K_C = k_C \sqrt{V_0}$

K_0 = standard cooling rate, about 7 W °C⁻¹ m⁻² for man resting in low air movement (Gagge, 1965)

V_0 = standard air movement rate

Equation (3-20) involves the skin temperature, T_S, because the equation describes the equivalent temperature at which a subject loses the same amount of heat at a standard cooling rate, K_0, as by radiation and convection in the original environment. Operative temperature can therefore be defined in terms of an imaginary environment having uniform air and radiant temperatures with which the subject can exchange the same total heat by radiation, convection, and conduction as he can in the actual complex environment.

Operative temperature is therefore a calorimetrically derived temperature scale that is inclusive for the nonevaporative or sensible modes of heat transfer but that does not take evaporative heat loss into account. A practical disadvantage in using the scale is that the mean skin temperature must be known.

Effective Radiant Flux

Gagge (1970) has described how the dry heat exchange between an organism and its environment can be considered in two parts.

1. The effective radiant flux. This is the heat flow by radiation caused only by surrounding surfaces radiating at temperatures different from air temperature.

2. The Newtonian heat flux. This is heat flow by radiation and convection to an imaginary environment uniformly at the same air temperature (with mean radiant temperature equal to air temperature) and with the same air movement as the original environment. The combined radiant–convective heat transfer coefficient determines the magnitude of this component.

The effective radiant flux is derived in the following manner. An equation to represent dry heat equilibrium, excluding conduction, can be written:

$$M_D = K_R(T_S - T_W) + K_C(T_S - T_A) \quad (3\text{--}21)$$

where M_D = metabolic rate less evaporative heat loss and less any external work done

T_S = mean skin temperature

This can be rearranged:

$$M_D + K_R(T_W - T_A) = K(T_S - T_A) \quad (3\text{--}22)$$

where $K = K_R + K_C$ and is the combined radiant–convective heat transfer coefficient.

The quantity $K(T_S - T_A)$ on the right-hand side of Eq. (3–22) represents the Newtonian heat loss in an imaginary environment in which T_A is both the air temperature and the mean radiant temperature. The term $K_R(T_W - T_A)$, on the lefthand side of the equation, is the effective radiant flux, and it is defined as the radiant energy exchange by an object of the same shape as the organism considered but having a surface temperature equal to the air temperature. When $T_W = T_A$, that is, when the air and mean radiant temperatures are equal, this quantity becomes zero. The greater the difference between the air and the mean radiant temperature, the larger is the effective radiant temperature, and the larger is the effective radiant flux (ERF). When $T_W > T_A$, ERF can be considered as a heat load added to M_D, to be dissipated as part of the radiant–convective transfer $K(T_S - T_A)$. If there is no conductive component, and the net radiant effect is a heat load, M_D plus the radiant heat load must be dissipated by convection if the heat balance is to be maintained. Evaporative heat loss from a sweating animal increases greatly under these conditions, and M_D becomes negative. However, evaporative loss from a nonsweating animal, such as the pig, under dry conditions is limited almost entirely to the respiratory component, and convective loss is relatively more important in thermoregulation. For this reason, cool floors that act as heat sinks and exogenous water for evaporative loss are of great practical importance for pig husbandry under hot conditions.

Gagge (1970) has pointed out that the ERF is the sum of each radiant field caused, for example, by a heated wall, a cold window, a heater, or the sun. The ERF is independent of the organism's surface temperature and of the temperature of its coat or of man's clothes. Gagge gives an account of methods of measuring ERF and of the uses to which it can be put in assessing the thermal environment.

Responses of Different Species to High Temperatures

Animals of different species have different ways of responding to high environmental temperatures. Man has considerable ability to sweat from the very large number of eccrine sweat glands distributed over the body surface. He thus produces a larger "percent wetted area" from which evaporation, and consequently cooling, can take place. Sweating is also quantitatively important in some animals, for example, the donkey and cattle, but for many other animals evaporative loss from the body surface plays only a minor role. This is true for the dog, sheep, and pig. The dog has a highly developed panting mechanism that permits a high rate of evaporative cooling from the upper respiratory tract without disturbance to the acid–base balance of the body fluids. Under hot conditions, the sheep and the pig both show a marked increase in respiratory rate and volume, but the evaporative cooling obtained in this way is not as great as in the dog. The pig has the added behavioral adaptation of wallowing in any water or mud that may be available. It thus provides itself with a highly effective wetted area for evaporative loss from exogenously derived water in the place of endogenously derived sweat.

Although these several species show dissimilarities in respect of the mechanisms of evaporative cooling they employ, they have in common the peripheral vasodilata- tion that accompanies environmental temperatures above the critical temperature. Vasodilatation in the poorly insulated parts of animals that have heavy insulation over a large part of the body is an important mechanism for heat dissipation. For example, heat loss from the poorly insulated limbs of sheep increases considerably with vasodilatation. In contrast, vasodilatation under the fleece covering the trunk has little effect on sensible heat transfer. The insulation of the fleece is so large that the decreased internal insulation makes relatively little difference to the total insulation. Adaptations of animals and man to hot environments are discussed in Chapters 9 and 10.

CHAPTER 4

Evaporative Heat Loss

Under hot conditions the amount of heat that can be lost through sensible channels is limited. Moreover, when the dry bulb temperature and the radiant temperature are above body temperature there is a net gain of heat. Evaporative heat loss therefore becomes progressively more important for the maintenance of body temperature as the ambient temperature rises. The vaporization of water from the body may take place (1) from the respiratory tract, where the rate may be increased in panting animals and (2) from the surface of the skin, where the loss falls into three categories: (a) water lost by diffusion through the skin and not subject to physiological control; (b) sweating from special glands, which is under physiological control; or (c) evaporation of moisture derived either from saliva or urine applied to the body surface by the animal or from wallowing in mud and water.

Although the physical basis for the amount of heat lost by evaporation of water is the same in each instance, the actual conditions under which the evaporation occurs may vary considerably depending on the site

of vaporization and the particular anatomy of the animals under consideration.

Evaporative Loss from the Respiratory Tract

When air is taken into the respiratory tract its temperature closely approximates that of the body and it becomes saturated, or very nearly so, with water vapor. When this air is expelled from the body its temperature may fall because the incoming air had a cooling effect on the tissues and a heat exchange system operates. The extent to which this happens varies both with the species and with the circumstances in which the animal finds itself. It is also possible that some dehumidification takes place before the air leaves the body; in the ox, McLean (1963b) has estimated that the expired air is sometimes only 90 percent saturated with water vapor. Several factors influence the extent to which heat and water exchange can occur.

1. The anatomical arrangement of the respiratory tract. Of particular importance is the ratio of the surface area of the heat and water exchange surfaces to the volume of space taken up by the air. A wide respiratory passage obviously allows relatively less air to contact the walls than a narrow one.
2. The air flow in the respiratory tract. If air flows through the passages too quickly heat and water vapor exchange may not be complete. If the flow is turbulent the exchange is processed faster than if it is laminar.
3. The blood flow to the moist surfaces. This factor influences the transfer of both heat and water to the exchange surface.

It is therefore of considerable importance to make detailed measurements on the particular animal in the particular circumstances before accurate measurements of heat loss from the respiratory tract can be made. Moreover, it cannot be assumed that the temperature and humidity of the inspired air is always the same as that of the general atmosphere in which the animal is placed. In man Lewis et al. (1969) have shown by means of schlieren photography that the inspired air is derived in part from a stream of air that rises along the front of the body. The very fact that this air stream can be detected by the schlieren technique means that it is at a temperature different from that of the general atmosphere, and because it has traveled over the body it may well be humidified. In other species, because of different anatomical arrangements, the inhaled air stream may not be preconditioned by the animal's own body. However, observation of a group of sleeping animals, such as rats or pigs, suggests that the inspired air may well be derived from a microclimate where both the dry bulb and wet bulb temperature differ from those of the atmosphere around the group. In the laboratory under strictly con-

trolled experimental conditions the humidity and temperature of both inspired and expired air may be accurately determined, but under more natural conditions this may not always be so and the possible resultant errors should be appreciated. The difference in volume between inspired and expired air is likely to be less than 1 percent and can therefore be neglected (McCutchan and Taylor, 1951).

As pointed out in Chapter 2, the total heat loss by panting is determined from the change in enthalpy. In some instances, however, interest centers not so much on total heat loss as on water loss and therefore the weights of water lost may be found (Chapters 1 and 2). When this quantity is known it is often useful to express it as milligrams water lost per liter of air breathed. In this way the relative efficiencies of animals in the conservation of water in hot climates can be compared. On the other hand, the efficiency of panting as a means of heat loss should be expressed as joules per liter of air breathed, using the change in enthalpy to make the calculation.

Conservation of Water Loss from the Respiratory Tract in a Hot Dry Climate

In hot desert regions the deployment of evaporative water loss in the control of body temperature is limited because of the restricted water supply and in some instances the accent shifts from thermoregulation to water conservation. Schmidt-Nielsen (1964) has made some calculations of the amount of heat that animals in desert climates absorb from the environment. This quantity depends on the surface area of the body available to absorb heat. Small animals, with their relatively large surface area to body weight ratio, tend to absorb relatively more heat than do large ones. His computations reveal that in given conditions under which an animal weighing 100 gm must evaporate water at the rate of 15 percent of its body weight per hour in order to keep in heat balance, an animal of only 10 gm must use water at the rate of 30 percent of its body weight. In the absence of a wallow such a high rate of water loss can hardly be sustained, and it is therefore not surprising to find that such small animals do not pant. Some data from various workers collected by Folk (1966) are given in Table 4–1, which illustrates the proportion of body weight that must be lost by different species in order to control body temperature in a hot dry climate.

Table 4–1. Percentage of Body Weight that Must Be Lost by Evaporation Per Hour to Maintain Body Temperature in a Hot Dry Climate of 40°C[a]

Species	Water evaporated as percentage of body weight
Mouse	21.5
Hamster	12.8
Rat	8.5
Rabbit	4.8
Dog	2.4
Man	1.5
Donkey	1.3
Camel	0.8

[a] From data collected from various sources by Folk (1966).

Studies of the kangaroo rat and other small mammals (Schmidt-Nielsen, 1964) have shown that the actual quantity of water lost from the respiratory tract is less than that to be expected if the temperature of the expired air is close to core temperature. In fact, the small diameter of the air passages facilitates heat exchange between the air and the passage surface and a countercurrent heat exchange system operates (Jackson and Schmidt-Nielsen, 1964). The water evaporated from the moist surface of the respiratory passage during inspiration reduces the temperature of the tissues. When the air is expelled it is cooled, its temperature falling

from core temperature to 25°C. The difference in the amount of vapor held by saturated air at 38°C and at 25°C is considerable and water is condensed on the respiratory passage to be evaporated again at the next inspiration (Fig. 4–1). The degree to which this exchange system operates varies between species, but the large surface area to volume ratio of the respiratory passages in small animals favors heat exchange in them. In man the expired air is near to 32°C at 20°C ambient temperature.

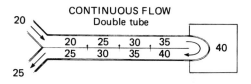

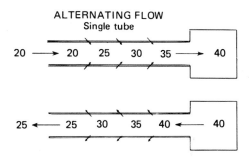

Fig. 4–1. Two types of heat exchange system. The lower system represents that in the respiratory tract, in which inspired air draws heat and water from the walls and gives both back again at expiration (Jackson and Schmidt-Nielsen, 1964).

Birds

The problem of conserving water loss in birds has received less attention, but it is known that in spite of the water taken up by air that is breathed in from the cold and then warmed to body temperature, water loss in birds remains fairly constant at low temperatures (Dawson and Hudson, 1970). Schmidt-Nielsen et al. (1969) have produced evidence demonstrating that a heat exchange system operates in small birds just as it does in small mammals. They have found that at ambient temperatures between 12°C and 30°C the exhaled air is 8°–25°C below body temperature.

water is thus used twice. The calculated percentage saving in water loss when the body temperature is 38°C and the relative humidity is 25 percent is 27, 10, and 4 percent at ambient temperatures of 30°C, 35°C, and 38°C, respectively.

Lizards

Lizards have also been shown to achieve economy of water loss through the respiratory tract. In at least one instance, this involves fairly complex adaptation. In the desert iguana Murrish and Schmidt-Nielsen (1970) have described how the secretion of the salt gland collects in a pouch near the opening of the nostril (Fig. 4–2). Inspired air passes over this pool and so is partly humidified by water that is already outside the body and which had to be excreted in order to eliminate the unwanted salt. The

Increased Evaporative Heat Loss from the Respiratory Tract during Panting

An increased ventilation rate, which is usually associated with an increased respiratory frequency, is employed widely among reptiles, birds, and mammals as a means of increasing respiratory heat loss. The terms "panting," "thermal polypnea," "tachypnea," and "hyperpnea" are all used to indicate the increased evaporative heat loss, but precise definitions have not always been

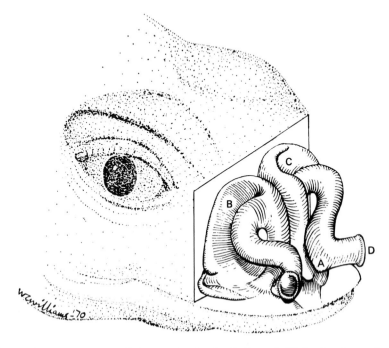

Fig. 4–2. Special arrangement of the nasal salt gland (B and C) in the desert iguana. Water already excreted from the body collects at the depression A to be used to humidify inspired air. The same water is in effect used twice by the iguana. D is the external opening (Murrish and Schmidt-Nielsen, 1970).

made. In some instances, "panting" may simply mean an increase in respiratory frequency, but in others the term is restricted to the type of breathing that occurs when the mouth is open.

Until recently, there has appeared little to choose among such definitions because each seemed to indicate a stage in the increase of evaporative heat loss. It has now been demonstrated in the dog, however (Schmidt-Nielsen et al., 1970), that the amount of water lost from the respiratory tract depends very largely on whether countercurrent heat exchange is allowed to take place in the respiratory tract. These workers have found that during normal breathing, when air enters and leaves via the nostril, the exhaled air is close to 28°C and the amount of heat lost is calculated to be 62 J/ liter. Under heat stress when the mouth is open, however, air enters through the nostrils and leaves via the mouth. This prevents heat exchange, with the result that the expired air is at 38°C and heat loss is 116 J/ liter. At very high rates of panting some air also enters via the mouth: but twice as much leaves. Open-mouthed panting thus approximately doubles the rate of heat loss, at least in the dog. Of course, this is not to say that an increased rate of ventilation with the mouth closed does not increase heat loss; it simply means that opening the mouth increases the efficiency, which, as is discussed below, is of importance in controlling the development of respiratory alkalosis.

It is not uncommon to find references to panting and evaporative heat loss from the lungs. The evidence is against there being any heat exchange in the lungs themselves, however, because the temperature of the blood in the pulmonary artery and in the carotid artery is the same. Bligh (1957a) and Mather et al. (1953) have found no evidence of cooling in the lung even when inspired air is at −18°C. The temperature of blood leaving the head via the jugular vein, which drains the upper respiratory tract, is on the other hand lower than that in the carotid artery. When evaporation is pre-vented by an increase in the humidity of the inspired air, this difference disappears until body temperature rises above the ambient temperature (Ingram and Whittow, 1962a) (Fig. 4–3). Heat loss is therefore most probably confined to the upper respiratory tract.

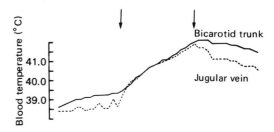

Fig. 4–3. The effect of preventing evaporative heat loss by increasing the humidity of the ambient air (at arrow on left). When the humidity rises, the difference in temperature between the blood and the carotid artery and the blood in the jugular vein is abolished until body temperature has increased to nearly 41.0°C. As soon as the humidity falls (arrow on right) the temperature difference is increased and the body temperature begins to fall (Ingram and Whittow, 1962b).

Pattern of Breathing: Respiratory Frequency and Tidal Volume

The measurement of respiratory frequency is relatively simple and may consist of only visually counting flank movements or of connecting some type of belt round the animal's body. Such devices are unlikely to impede breathing and the results are not likely to be subject to much error. The measurement of tidal volume, however involves more complicated apparatus, such as a face mask either incorporating a pneumotachograph or connected to a spirometer. The animal must be trained to wear such a mask, and it presents some resistance to air flow. Alternatively, the animal can be enclosed in a whole body plethsmograph, but such a device must be free of leaks and obviously restricts the animal's movements. The limitations of these methods have been pointed out by Richards (1970), in his review of the biology of thermal panting, and must be appreciated in interpreting the results obtained.

The pattern of breathing seen during the development of panting, however, involves differences between species that cannot be related purely to differences in the techniques used to study them. Hemingway (1938), among others, has described how the frequency of breathing increases abruptly and tidal volume declines when the dog is exposed to heat. In spite of this decline in the amount of air taken at each breath, however, the minute volume (frequency × tidal volume) increases. The change in breathing pattern has been shown by Crawford (1962) to involve a switch in respiratory frequency to the resonant frequency of the respiratory system. He found that his dogs panted at a frequency of 5.33 ± 0.7 cycles/second and that the natural frequency of the respiratory system was 5.28 ± 0.3 cycles/second. The saving in energy achieved by taking advantage of the natural rebound of the system is quite large. Using the formula developed by Otis et al. (1950) to calculate the work of breathing in men, Crawford has concluded that if the dog were to pant at any other frequency the extra heat generated would be expected to offset the heat loss by evaporation.

This demonstration reveals a remarkable economy on the part of the physiological system and there has been a tendency to believe that all panting animals behave in the same way. However, observation shows that this is not invariably true. In the ox (Beakley and Findlay, 1955; Kleiber and Regan, 1933), respiratory frequency increases stepwise with each increase in environmental temperature and may reach a steady state at any value. For example, at ambient temperatures of 15°–20°C respiratory frequency increases by three per minute-degree centigrade and above 25°C at six per minute-degree centigrade. Similarly, Findlay and Ingram (1961) have shown that if a constant

radiant heat load is imposed on cattle at different environmental temperatures below the critical temperature, the respiratory frequency stabilizes at different levels. The sheep resembles the dog more than the ox in that the range of ambient temperatures over which intermediate respiratory frequencies are observed is small. The cat (Robinson and Lee, 1941) and the pig (Ingram, 1964a) likewise display a fairly steep rise in respiratory frequency with increases in ambient temperature, although intermediate frequencies are possible. The rabbit, however, according to the figures published by Lee et al. (1941), shows a response resembling that seen in cattle (Figs. 4–4 and 4–5).

Because the tidal volume falls when panting begins some of the increased volume of air washes back and forth in the respiratory deadspace, rather than in the lungs (Hales and Webster, 1967; Hales and Findlay, 1968a), which is of importance in limiting the development of respiratory alkalosis. Under very severe heat stress, however, most animals change their pattern of panting a second time. The frequency reaches a high value and then falls slightly at the same time as the tidal volume increases (Fig. 4–6). This type of respiration, which is sometimes called "second-phase" breathing, has been described in detail for the ox by Findlay (1954) and for the sheep by Hales and Webster (1967). Its significance is not fully understood, but it does result in a further increase in minute volume. The pig appears to be exceptional in that unequivocal second-phase breathing does not occur, at least not in the young animal (Ingram and Legge, 1969). In this species, however, when body temperature is between 42°C and 43°C, there is a very slight increase in tidal volume, although respiratory frequency remains the same. The difference between the pig and other animals in this respect may therefore be more one of degree than of kind.

Birds have no sweat glands and therefore depend very largely on panting as a means of controlled evaporative heat loss. This subject has been covered in recent re-

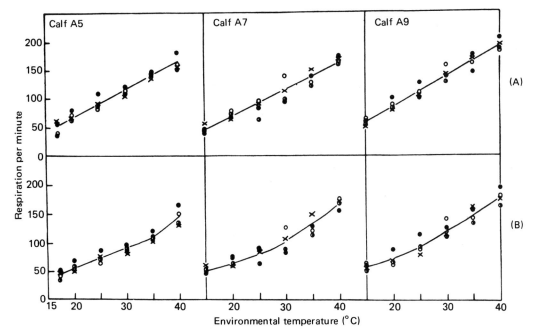

Fig. 4–4. The relation between respiratory frequency and environmental temperature in cattle. (A) The maximum or peak frequency; (B) the frequency after 6 hours. ○, ●, X refer to separate experiments (Beakley and Findlay, 1955).

views by Salt (1964) and Richards (1970). The maximum rate of panting varies considerably between species but very high rates, up to 700 a minute, have been recorded. As in mammals the development of panting falls broadly into two groups (Dawson and Hudson, 1970). In one group, including the domestic fowl (Hutchinson, 1955) and the house sparrow, the respiratory frequency increases gradually as ambient temperature increases. In the other, including the ostrich (Schmidt-Nielsen et al. 1969) and the rock dove (Calder and Schmidt-Nielsen, 1966), the frequency changes abruptly, as in the dog. In some of the latter instances a saving in energy expenditure may be achieved if panting occurs at the natural resonant frequency of the respiratory system but in the ostrich, at least, this does not appear to be so (Schmidt-Nielsen et al. 1969).

In addition to panting, which involves taking air deep into the respiratory system, some (but not all) birds also employ a process known as "gular flutter." The rapid flexing of the hyoid apparatus moves the loose skin of the throat or gular region, which is well vascularized, and draws air over its moist surface and heat loss is augmented. Rates of gular flutter vary from 70 to 1000 a minute and in most species seem to be independent of heat load; the evaporative loss is controlled by intermittent activity. In other species, however, the rate of flutter increases with the rise of ambient temperature. Dawson and Hudson (1970) have collected information form a number of sources. They point out that in some cases the rate of flutter is the same as the respiratory frequency, for example, in the roadrunner (Calder and Schmidt-Nielsen, 1967) whereas in others, for example, cormorants (Bartholomew et al., 1968), the two are independent, the gular flutter being at the higher frequency. In some birds, for example, the poorwill, gular flutter occurs in the absence of panting. The flutter may occur at the resonant frequency of the system and then less energy expenditure is required to achieve a given water loss than is required by panting.

The problems associated with panting

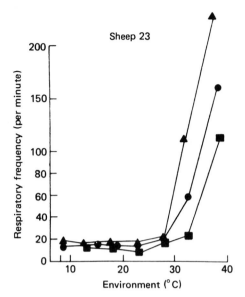

Fig. 4–5. Changes in respiratory frequency in sheep as environmental temperature changes. The animal was fed on low (■), medium (●), and high (▲) planes of nutrition (Blaxter et al., 1959).

in birds are further complicated by the presence of air sacs as well as lungs. The general arrangement of the air sac system is shown in Fig. 4–7. The relatively small and inelastic lungs make connections with the sacs, which extend widely over the body. A simplified version is shown in Fig. 4–8, where the anterior and posterior air sacs have been grouped together. There has been considerable debate over how air flows in this system, and for a detailed account the reader should consult Salt and Zeuthen (1960), Salt (1964), and King and Farner (1964). Recent work by Bretz and Schmidt-Nielsen (1970) favors the view that, on inspiration, air passes straight down into the posterior sacs via the mesobronchus and, at the same time, from the lung via the parabronchi to the anterior sacs. At expiration, air passes from the posterior sacs via the parabronchi to the lungs and from the anterior sacs to the exterior.

The extent to which the air sacs are filled, however, can be varied independently of lung ventilation, as has been indicated in

studies by Calder and Schmidt-Nielsen (1966) on the rock dove. In this species respiratory frequency does not change when the ambient temperature increases from 30°C to 40°C but the minute volume increases by a

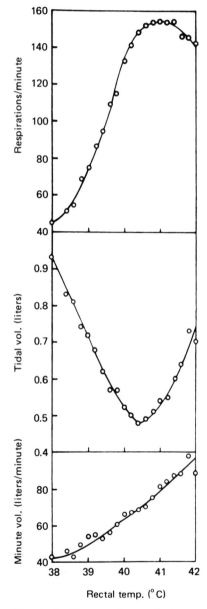

Fig. 4–6. Changes in respiratory pattern as body temperature increases in cattle. Note the change in tidal volume and respiratory frequency at a rectal temperature of 40.5°C (Findlay, 1957).

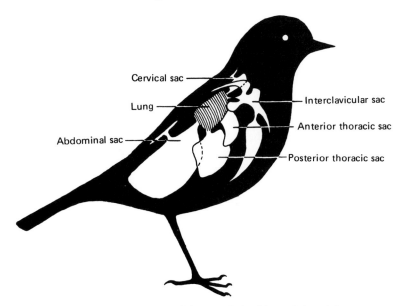

Fig. **4–7.** General layout of air sacs and lungs of the bird (Salt, 1964).

factor of almost four. The tidal volume must therefore also increase fourfold, although there is no indication from the blood chemistry that pulmonary ventilation also increases. The implication is that the increased tidal volume is accounted for by ventilation of the air sacs rather than of the lung itself. According to Salt (1964), it is probably the anterior sacs that function in this way. Above 40°C, the respiratory frequency increases in the rock dove, gular flutter begins, and the total ventilation is increased still further, but during this phase tidal volume decreases. If ambient temperature is increased still more, minute volume continues to rise while respiratory frequency and gular flutter continue at the same rate. At this point, however, pulmonary ventilation must also increase because the blood pH rises.

The changes in pattern of breathing in the domestic fowl (Hutchinson, 1955) follow a different course. In this species respiration increases in step with increases in ambient temperature; tidal volume decreases and minute volume rises (Frankel et al., 1962). Under very severe heat stress there is a secondary decline in frequency and an increase in tidal volume, similar to that seen in mammals, with a resultant further in-

crease in minute volume (Randall and Hiesland, 1939; Stein et al., 1964). For a more detailed discussion of the differences between different species of birds the reader is re-

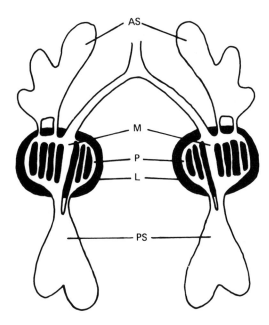

Fig. **4–8.** Diagram of lungs and air sacs in the bird. AS, anterior sacs; P, parabronchi; PS, posterior sacs; M, mesobronchus; L, lung tissue.

ferred to the specialized reviews of the subject by Salt (1964), King and Farner (1964), Richards (1970), and Dawson and Hudson (1970).

Reptiles Many reptiles live in desert regions and, as Templeton (1970) points out, they may employ evaporative heat loss only as an emergency measure for relatively short periods. In any event, the respiratory frequency is temperature-dependent in all reptiles, although some species do exhibit a greater increase than others and may therefore be said to pant. In heliothermic lizards and collared lizards, there is a coincident decline in tidal volume when panting begins, although in the collared lizard Dawson and Templeton (1963) have found that evaporative loss increases at a body temperature 2°C below that at which an increased respiratory frequency is apparent. The heliothermic lizards display the most highly developed form of panting; the mouth is open and the highly vascularized tongue is extended (Figs. 4–9 and 4–10).

Efficiency of Panting

One measure of the efficiency of panting is the percentage of the total heat production it can dissipate. This quantity obviously depends on the humidity of the inspired air, for the more water it contains the less can be added to a given volume at a given temperature. For any humidity, however, more water can be lost at higher temperatures. The rise in body temperature during heat stress is thus an aid to heat loss. Against this, a rise in body temperature also results in a rise in heat production because of the Arrhenius-Van't Hoff effect. Moreover, the very effort of panting involves work and therefore heat production, and panting that can dissipate very little more heat than it generates is clearly very inefficient. Unfortunately, different animals have been studied under a variety of conditions and using several techniques, so comparisons are difficult to make with precision. Furthermore, some animals sweat as well as pant.

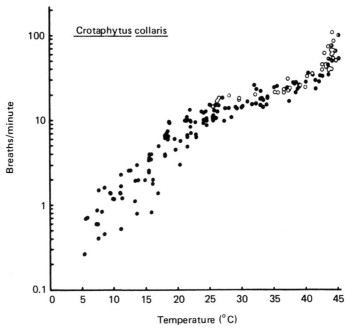

Fig. 4–9. Relation between respiratory frequency and body temperature in the collared lizard (Templeton and Dawson, 1963; copyright University of Chicago).

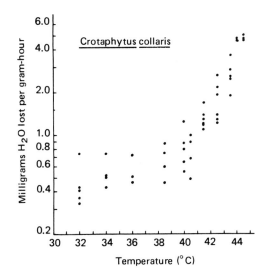

Fig. 4–10. Increased water loss in the collared lizard at high ambient temperatures (Dawson and Templeton, 1963; copyright University of Chicago).

The principal channel of evaporative loss in dogs is by panting. Dogs can accompany man in the desert, and their efficient system of panting is underlined by the very old experiment by Dr. Blagden, mentioned in Chapter 1. The cat, as judged by its tolerance of a hot climate, probably pants with an efficiency similar to that of the dog (Robinson and Lee, 1941), although the fact that the cat licks its fur under heat stress complicates the comparison. The rabbit is reported to have no sweat glands, but water loss from the skin is high (Keeton, 1924). It probably loses less than half of its evaporative heat via the respiratory system under moderate conditions and even less under severe stress (Johnson et al., 1958). The sheep is capable of a considerable increase in minute volume, 5.5 times the resting value (Hales and Webster, 1967). Rick et al. (1950) believed the increase to be 12-fold, but their peak minute volume was similar to that found by Hales and Webster. The actual percentage of the total heat production lost by panting in the sheep, however, varies between 11 and 40 percent, depending on the length of the fleece, which limits cutaneous heat loss (Brockway et al., 1965). In the view of Lee

and Robinson (1941), who studied a number of animals under similar conditions, the sheep displays a high degree of heat tolerance that is partly a reflection of its capacity to pant. The ox depends on both panting and sweating to evaporate water; McLean (1963b) concluded that sweating was the major means of heat loss when the animal is subjected to heat stress. The pig, which does not sweat, tolerates heat poorly if it is not allowed to wallow and is capable of dissipating only a relatively small proportion of its heat production by panting (Ingram and Legge, 1969).

The differences among animals make comparisons of panting abilities impossible unless some common basis can be established. One such basis is the energy cost of panting compared with the amount of extra air taken through the system. In order for this determination to be made the rise in oxygen consumption with increase in ambient temperature must be found under conditions that do not excite the animal to struggle. The increased oxygen consumption must then be partitioned into (1) that from the Arrhenius-Van't Hoff effect, that is, the increase caused by a chemical reaction proceeding faster at higher temperatures, and (2) that from the additional muscular effect of panting. The value given to the first of these parts depends largely on the value of the Q_{10}. Most living systems seem to have a Q_{10} of 2; that is, the rate doubles when there is a 10°C increase in temperature, but departure from this value can be marked. The second portion (2) is assumed to be chiefly from the work of breathing but should also include, for example, any extra energy expenditure by the heart as cardiac output also tends to rise with increases in body temperature.

In the ox, Whittow and Findlay (1968) and Hales and Findlay (1968a) have estimated the cost of rapid shallow breathing to be 0.5 ml O_2 per liter, which is a figure similar to that in nonpanting man (Otis, 1954). At high body temperatures, however, this value increases to 1.2 ml O_2 per liter. Pigs have been estimated to use 1.4 ml O_2 per liter of breathed air at body temperatures up to 40.5°C, but above this temperature the animals become restless and estimates can no longer be made (Ingram and Legge, 1969) (Fig. 4–11). The oxygen cost of panting in the dog has also been estimated at between 1.2 and 1.6 ml O_2 per liter of air breathed, in spite of the evidence that this species pants at its resonant frequency. As mentioned, the figure calculated is much influenced by the value used for the Q_{10}. Nevertheless, it seems unlikely that panting is expensive in terms of heat production.

Birds

Because no birds have been reported to have sweat glands, the capacity of respiratory evaporative water loss to dissipate the metabolic heat is easier to compute. The

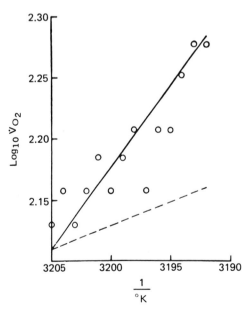

Fig. 4–11. Relation between log of the rate of oxygen consumption and the reciprocal of body temperature on the absolute scale. The dotted line indicates the theoretical relationship assuming a Q_{10} of 2. The difference between the dotted line and the continuous line represents the additional oxygen consumption associated with panting (Ingram and Legge, 1969).

most efficient bird seems to be the poorwill (Bartholomew et al., 1962), which chiefly because of its low metabolic rate can lose over 160 percent of its heat production by this channel. The red-breasted nuthatch can lose 70 percent of its metabolic heat by panting when the ambient temperature is close to body temperature (Mugass and Templeton, 1970). Other birds also have been demonstrated to be capable of withstanding ambient temperatures above their body temperature (Lasiewski et al., 1966; Calder and Schmidt-Nielsen, 1967; Crawford and Schmidt-Nielsen, 1967) and birds must therefore be regarded as efficient panters.

Reptiles

Templeton (1960) and Dawson and Templeton (1963, 1966) have shown that the desert iguana can dissipate its heat production at an ambient temperature of 44°C, and the collared lizard more than its heat production at 44°C. The panting alligator lizard on the other hand can lose only 60 percent of its metabolic heat by this channel at 38°C.

Panting and Its Effect on Blood Gases

The increase in ventilation rate during panting not only increases the loss of water but also changes the gas composition of the blood by washing out the CO_2. This effect is to some extent offset by the fact that the increased ventilation rate is largely restricted to the respiratory dead space. But an increased alveolar ventilation also occurs, particularly during second-phase breathing. The consequence of this is a loss of CO_2, and a rise in blood pH (alkalosis) of an order that is likely to result in severe tetany and death in a nonpanting animal, such as man.

In the initial stages of panting, pCO_2 and pH are hardly changed in the ox and sheep. When body temperature increases and the slower deeper breathing begins, however, pCO_2 falls steadily to below 10 mm Hg and pH may rise above 7.8 (Hales and Findlay, 1968b; Bianca and Findlay, 1962, in the ox; Hales and Webster, 1967, in sheep). In birds, because of the different anatomical arrangement, some increase in total ventilation rate can take place without any great change in the ventilation of the lungs (Calder and Schmidt-Nielsen, 1966). During second-phase breathing, however, there is nevertheless a fall in pCO_2 and a consequent rise in pH. On exposure to moderate heat Mueller (1966) found only a small shift in pH in the domestic fowl. During second-phase breathing Frankel and Frascella (1968) obtained values of 11 mm Hg for pCO_2 and 7.66 for pH. In the pigeon, under severe heat stress, the values were 8 mm Hg and 7.79 (Calder and Schmidt-Nielsen, 1966), although birds tend to have lower resting values of pCO_2 than do mammals. In spite of the large change in pH, symptoms of tetany are not displayed in panting animals except under the most severe conditions (Hales and Findlay, 1968a).

Panting does not appear to alter the pCO_2 (Findlay and Whittow, 1966) unless body temperature is very high and the change to second-phase breathing cannot be attributed to hypoxia (Hales and Findlay, 1968b).

Mechanisms that Control Panting

The problems associated with the control of panting have been reviewed by Richards (1970) and form part of the wider issue of the control of thermoregulatory mechanisms in general. This has received attention by Hardy (1961), Bligh (1966, 1973), and Hammel (1968). For many years the problem was seen as one of deciding whether animals responded to a change in the deep body temperature or to the temperature at the periphery. It has recently become apparent, however, that stimuli from a number of regions interact with each other in the control of panting. Local heating of the preoptic region of the hypothalamus is accompanied by a rise in respiratory frequency in panting animals, as demonstrated by Barbour (1912), among others, and as has since been confirmed by Magoun et al. (1938) in the cat, Anderson et al. (1956) in the goat, and Fusco et al. (1961) in the dog. The ambient temperature at which the local heating is carried out in conscious animals, however, modifies the response. The magnitude of the increase in respiratory frequency is reduced at low temperature (Ingram and Whittow, 1962) in the ox. In the pig, no increase in respiratory frequency is observed in response to heating the hypothalamus at ambient temperatures below the critical temperature (Baldwin and Ingram, 1968). Cooling the hypothalamic region arrests panting.

In addition to the preoptic region of the hypothalamus the cervical region of the spinal cord also influences panting and other thermoregulatory mechanisms (Jessen, 1967). This effect is mediated through the hypothalamus (Kosaka et al., 1969), however, and the magnitude of the change in respiratory frequency in response to a given change in spinal temperature depends on peripheral temperature (Ingram and Legge, 1971). Other regions deep in the body have also been demonstrated particularly sensitive to temperature changes and implicated in the control of panting; for example, the abdomen of sheep (Rawson and Quick, 1970), the wall of the vena cava (Bligh, 1961), and some nonspecified regions in the rabbit (Guieu and Hardy, 1970a). Heating and cooling parts of the medulla have also been shown to affect respiration but the significance of temperature receptors in this region is in doubt and they probably play no part under normal circumstances (Chai and Wang, 1970).

There is also a large body of evidence demonstrating the importance of peripheral receptors in the control of thermal panting. Several experiments have shown that panting can occur in the absence of any change in deep body temperature as, for example, when the humidity is increased (Bligh, 1957b) or when an animal is exposed to radiant heat (Findlay and Ingram, 1961). Perhaps the most dramatic demonstration of the effect of peripheral receptors in the initiation of panting is that by Waites (1962), who warmed the scrotum of the ram and observed panting that persisted in spite of a fall of 2°C in body temperature.

The control of panting in mammals therefore appears to depend on the interaction of signals from a number of points, both deep in the body and at the periphery. This view is supported by the studies of Chatonnet et al. (1964), who controlled skin temperature in the dog by immersion in a water bath and found that panting occurred in response only to certain combinations of deep body and peripheral temperature. Ingram and Legge (1971) obtained similar results in the pig in an experiment in which regions of the skin were held at different temperatures by means of a controlled-temperature coat and deep body receptors were stimulated with implanted thermodes.

With respect to birds, in contrast, Richards (1970) concluded that panting was not established in domestic fowls unless body temperature increases. Peripheral stimuli alone did not appear to be sufficient, although they could facilitate or inhibit panting. However, birds have received less attention than mammals and a more definite statement must await the results of further work.

Evaporative Loss from the Skin by Passive Transfer of Water

Water may be lost through the skin in the absence of sweat glands, even at tem-peratures below the critical temperature, simply because skin is not completely impervious to water. Moreover, because the rate of water loss through the skin depends partly on the surface temperature of the epidermis, moisture vaporization increases when an animal vasodilates in response to heat. At thermoneutral and low ambient temperatures the rate of loss by this channel is of the order of 10 gm m^{-2} hr^{-1} in a wide variety of species, including man, and rises to about 30 gm m^{-2} hr^{-1} in a warm environment. In a sweating species, this loss is only a small proportion of the total, but in a species that does not sweat the contribution to heat loss is not unimportant.

Another factor governing the passive transfer of water through the skin is the vapor pressure of the air. Buettner (1953) has shown that under conditions of high humidity water vapor may pass into the body of a man from the environment. In pigs, which do not sweat, the passage of moisture vapor into the animal at high temperatures and humidities leads to an actual net gain of water (Ingram, 1965a).

Sweating

Sweat glands, until recently, have been classified as apocrine or eccrine on the basis of morphological and physiological criteria. The apocrine gland was believed to produce its secretion by a process known as necrobiosis. According to the original description, the cells lining the gland form protoplasmic protuberances, which extend into the lumen and finally become detached. Once free in the lumen of the gland these globules were believed to form a fluid, while the cells lining the gland, which had become flattened, began to grow again. The eccrine glands, in contrast, were thought to derive their contents from a process of secretion involving some sort of physiological pump.

In addition to this physiological division, the same names have been attached to glands largely for anatomical reasons. The apocrine gland is thus associated with a hair follicle and the eccrine gland is free. Yet another distinction between these two types of gland that has sometimes been made concerns the mode by which their contents are extruded onto the surface. The apocrine glands are invested with a distinct myoepithelium, which is believed to contract and force the luminal contents outward, like toothpaste out of a tube, whereas the eccrine glands are thought to depend on the pressure of secretion to expel the fluid.

The validity of the rigid distinction between the two types of sweat gland has been called into question by Weiner and Hellman (1960) in their comprehensive review of sweat glands, and also by Jenkinson (1967) and Bligh (1967). From these reviews it is clear that there is a wide variety of sweat glands and that the processes of sweat secretion and expulsion do not completely lend themselves to the above type of division. An alternative classification has now been suggested, the glands being described as epitrichial when associated with a hair follicle and atrichial when they are not associated with a hair follicle (Bligh, 1967). Although in practice this classification may usually amount to calling apocrine glands "epitrichial" and eccrine glands "atrichial," the new terms are free of any implied description of their mode of secretion and are therefore to be recommended.

Atrichial Glands (Eccrine)

The general body surface of man is richly supplied with atrichial glands. In the majority of cases the term "eccrine" refers to this type of gland, although much experimental work has been done on the glands in the cat's paw. In both instances the secretory part is a close coil, and the duct usually spirals to the skin surface. The lining epithelium is composed of both large and small cells (Montagna, 1956) that have sometimes been regarded as forming two layers. The cells contain both acidophilic and basophilic granules that are believed by some (Montagna, 1956) to be secretory. However, Shelley and Mescon (1952) maintain that in man, at least, there are no secretory granules. Nevertheless, it has been shown (Cormia and Kuykendall, 1955) that secretory activity does in fact involve the loss of some granular substance, for the number of clear cells has been observed to increase after secretory activity is stimulated. The cells lining the gland exhibit morphological changes after prolonged stimulation, becoming smaller and flattened, and it is possible that the different types of cell described in the sweat gland are in reality simply cells in different stages of exhaustion. During a nonsevere heat stimulus, however, Shelley and Mescon (1952) have found no gross change in the human sweat gland except a diminution in the amount of glycogen.

Epitrichial Glands (Apocrine)

Epitrichial glands have been described in most species, although their function may differ considerably both between species and, within the same animal, according to their location. In man, glands of this type are found in the axillae and do not become active until puberty; in other animals, for example cattle, their development does not appear to be associated with sexual maturation. The morphology of the glands has also been found subject to considerable variation between species, but the differences do not appear to give any clue to the gland's thermoregulatory role. In man, the glands associated with hair follicles are much larger than the rest and this has given rise to the generalization that "apocrine" glands are larger than "eccrine" glands. In fact the epitrichial glands of the ox are smaller than the atrichial glands of man.

The secretory part of the epitrichial gland may be saclike, as in the ox, goat, and sheep, but in other species, possibly the majority, it is a coiled structure (e.g., human axillae, horse, dog, monkey, pig). The duct usually takes a fairly straight course to the surface and is narrower than the secretory part. The opening may be near to where the hair follicle reaches the skin surface or some distance away.

The mode of secretion of these glands, as mentioned, was the subject of some dispute. The original description of the necrobiotic secretory cycle was based on descriptions of the epitrichial glands of man and it was supposed that a series of histological preparations showing "blebs" of cell content bulging from the cells or apparently free in the lumen of the gland represented stages of the secretory process.

Montagna (1956) and Kuno (1956) have cast doubts on this interpretation and there has been much recent evidence (see review by Jenkinson, 1967) to support them. Modern descriptions of the secretory cells agree on the presence of protuberances from the apical free border. Within the cell, the granules near the base are large; they become smaller near the apical surface, where vacuoles are also present. This arrangement has led to the idea that the secretory material is derived from the dissolution of the granules to form a clear liquid that is pinched off into the lumen of the gland. The secretory granules are not normally found within the lumen of the gland, however, and any rupturing of the membrane that allows them into the lumen is now thought to be an artifact produced during histological preparation. The likelihood is that the secretory process of these glands involves a combination of the pumping of fluid and the "pinching off" of minute cellular protuberances containing clear fluid. Moreover, the extent to which these processes contribute to the func-

tion of the gland probably varies considerably among species.

Numbers of Sweat Glands

The number of sweat glands in man varies both with the region of the body and between individuals. The highest density is in the palm of the hand and sole of the foot at 2000 per square centimeter; the face has 200–300 per square centimeter and the limbs and trunk have 100–200. Similar detailed studies are available for only a few other species. In the gorilla, there is a similar high density in the sole of the foot and hand, but absolute numbers are not available. In the chimpanzee the glands are said to be sparsely distributed. In cattle, Findlay and Yang (1951) have found 1000 per square centimeter on the lower limbs, 2000 on the trunk, and about 2500 on the neck, giving an average of about 1800 per square centimeter, compared with only 80–200 per square centimeter in man. The buffalo has only about 180 per square centimeter and the sheep has 240–340.

The density in young animals is greater than in the adult in both man and cattle.

Nature of the Substance Secreted

A number of techniques have been used to collect sweat, particularly in man (Robinson and Robinson, 1954). The whole body can be washed down with distilled water; the sweat can be absorbed onto pads or filter paper; the sweat can be allowed to collect in a large plastic bag covering a limb, or even the whole body. In the large axillary epitrichial glands of man, Shelley and Hurley (1952) have succeeded in inserting a 150μm glass capillary tube into the duct.

In methods involving the washing of the whole body, the original amounts of fluid secreted can be estimated from the weight loss of the subject after a suitable correction has been made for respiratory and metabolic weight losses. The resultant fluid represents only the average composition from glands all over the body. However, other methods using a plastic bag over the arm have been found to yield results that overestimate the concentration of solutes (Van Heyningen and Weiner, 1952), probably because under conditions of high humidity water is reabsorbed through the skin (Buettner, 1953). Methods involving the use of a pad probably do not suffer from this disadvantage and do allow the sweat composition of different regions to be compared. All the methods except those involving pipets directly from the duct, however, involve errors associated with the possible contamination of sweat with the secretion of the sebaceous glands.

Reviews of the literature on the composition of sweat are available in Rothman (1954), Robinson and Robinson (1954), and Kuno (1956), but most of the data refer to man. Human sweat produced on thermal stimulation is hypotonic to blood, and depletion of body water therefore proceeds faster than does depletion of electrolytes. It also follows from this that the production of sweat does not take place by simple diffusion alone.

The main solute is sodium chloride, but there is some disparity in the concentrations found by various investigators. Figures of between 200 and 400 mg percent have been published, but part of the differences may be related to the method of collection and the duration over which the samples were taken. The concentration of chloride rises as the rate of sweating increases. A rise in salt concentration has also been correlated with a rise in environmental temperature and also with an increase in skin temperature. After a period of acclimatization to a hot climate, there is a tendency for salt concentration to fall. This decline has been shown to depend on a fall in the salt reserves of the body because if sufficient extra salt is taken during the acclimatization period the decline in the amount of salt secreted does not occur. Similarly, if the salt content of the diet is reduced the amount present in sweat falls within a few days (Weiner and van Heyningen, 1952).

As mentioned in Chapter 6, it has been shown that during heat exposure the output of aldosterone increases (Hellmann et al., 1956). In spite of this the loss of salt during work at high temperatures may be sufficient to cause "heat cramp," and for efficient working it is necessary to provide not only adequate drinking water but also salt tablets (Haldane, 1929). Sweat from the palmar region may differ in composition from that produced over the general body surface, but as sweating on the palm of the hand decreases on exposure to heat and has no thermoregulatory function it is not considered here.

The concentration of urea in sweat is about twice as high as in blood. For this reason, sweating can be regarded to a very limited extent as an excretory process that takes over from the kidney during heat stress, when the volume of urine is reduced. It must be emphasized, however, that the amount of urea excreted in sweat is only a small fraction of the total excreted by the body. Lactic acid is present in sweat at a greater concentration than in plasma, and it is this which gives the sweat an acid pH. Other substances found in sweat are potassium, calcium, and traces of magnesium, phosphorus, copper, manganese, iron, and sulfates.

The chemical composition of the secretion of the epitrichial glands is less well documented. In the human, Shelley and Hurley (1953) have found reducing sugar, protein, ammonia, and iron. Protein has also been found in the epitrichial gland secretion of the horse and ox, but no iron has been detected. Glycogen has been reported to occur in the sweat glands of horses (Evans et al., 1957) and cattle (Yang, 1952). This probably gives rise to the small quantities of lactic acid that have been detected, although none is apparently present in axillary glands. In some species, odoriferous substances and pigments are also present, but in these instances the glands may not perform any thermoregulatory function.

Production of Sweat

The facts that sweat is hypotonic to plasma and that the amount of salt present depends on the salt content of the body point to some mechanism in the sweat gland involving active secretion or reabsorption. Processes of this kind require energy expenditure and it is possible that this is supplied by the conversion of glycogen to lactate. As Weiner and Hellmann (1960) point out, however, in order to show that this is indeed the case it is first necessary to demonstrate that lactate is synthesized in the gland and not simply removed from the plasma. Both points of view have been held, but Weiner and Hellmann (1960) believe that the lactate is formed in the gland. Their theory accounts for the presence of glycogen in the gland but not in the sweat and satisfies the energy requirements for the production of dilute sweat. Alternatively, it is possible that the lactate may simply be the product of anaerobic metabolism because its concentration increases when the blood supply is reduced.

The urea in sweat may also be formed in the gland as the result of metabolism, but it seems more probable that the high concentration is the result of water being reabsorbed (Schwartz et al., 1953). The duct of the human atrichial gland is well supplied with blood vessels, which makes it anatomically suitable as a site for water absorption. However, such absorption has not yet been demonstrated.

Expulsion of Sweat

Both types of gland are enveloped in a myoepithelium, which is rather more obvious in the epitrichial glands. Hurley and Shelley (1954) have found by direct observation that contraction of this muscle layer in the axillary gland expels fluid, and there is evidence, as discussed below, that this is true of several species. The atrichial glands in man and on the cat's paw, however, appear to secrete simply by overflow of the contents. Contraction of the myoepithelium, if it occurs, has very little effect.

It has recently become obvious that a similar overflow of contents also occurs in some epitrichial glands. Allen and Bligh (1969) have presented evidence demonstrating that there are differences among species in the relative contribution to the expulsion of fluid made by overflow and myoepithelium contraction. These authors have measured the rate of sweating using a ventilated capsule (McLean, 1963a). They have found that in the llama exposed to a high temperature water loss increases and thereafter there is a continuous steady loss of water. In the horse and donkey, the discharge is usually smooth but sometimes exhibits synchronous peaks of discharge. The ox displays a stepwise increase in moisture loss on initial exposure and thereafter a series of brief increments in water loss superimposed on a steady flow of moisture. Sheep and goats showed not a steady flow but a series of synchronous discharges from various points on the surface (Fig. 4–12). Allen and Bligh (1969) interpret their results as demonstrating that in such a species as the ox there is a continuous outpouring of sweat, because of simple overflowing of the glands, and also a periodic contraction of the myoepithelium. The llama, however, relies purely on an overflow and the sheep only on myoepithelial contraction. They support this conclusion by demonstrating that when the myoepithelium is caused to contract experimen-

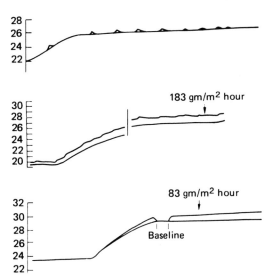

Fig. 4–12. The rate of moisture vaporization from the skin measured by the ventilated capsule technique. The upper trace in each case gives the wet bulb temperature of air that has passed through a capsule on the skin, and the lower trace gives the wet bulb temperature of room air. The difference between the two indicates the water loss through the skin. Top record, sheep; middle, cow; bottom, llama. In the trace for the llama a check on the baseline has been made by letting both wet bulbs sample room air (Allen and Bligh, 1969).

tally after an injection of adrenaline, similar peaks of sweat production occur. Synchronous fluctuations in sweat rate over different areas have also been reported in man (Custance, 1962), but there is disagreement over whether they relate to different numbers of glands being active or to myoepithelial activity.

Mechanisms that Control Sweating

On general theoretical grounds the sweat glands may be expected to depend on nervous stimulation or on some blood-borne agent, or possibly on some combination of these, in which a neurohumeral substance is released near the gland after nervous stimulation. Studies of nerve endings in tissue have been made with a view to determining whether the secretory epithelium is innervated, but the conclusions are not clearcut. In the atrichial glands of man and the cat, the earlier studies suggest that the nerve endings penetrate the glandular cells, but more recent studies have not confirmed this (Hellmann, 1955). In the epitrichial glands of the sheep, goat, and ox, Jenkinson and Blackburn (1967) and Jenkinson et al. (1966) have found no evidence of a nerve supply ending on the secretory cells, nor has one been demonstrated in the axillary glands in man.

An alternative approach to the study of mechanisms by which sweat glands are stimulated is to search for the presence of the enzymes that destroy acetylcholine or noradrenaline. Such investigations must be approached with caution however, because failure to demonstrate the presence of cholinesterase does not necessarily mean that the nerves are not cholinergic. Hellmann (1955) has found that the atrichial glands of man, cat, monkey, and rat contain specific cholinesterase but do not contain monoamine oxidase. The epitrichial glands of the horse (Hellmann, 1955) contain no cholinesterase but do contain monoamine oxidase. The sweat glands of sheep, goat, ox, and pig also contain monoamine oxidase, and some specific and nonspecific cholinesterase has been found as well.

Experiments involving the injection of adrenergic and cholinergic drugs and their specific inhibitors in general strengthen the idea that atrichial glands are cholinergic and epitrichial glands adrenergic. At least, in man, however, intradermal injections of adrenaline can cause sweating, although because agents that block the action of adrenaline do not prevent thermal sweating it is unlikely that adrenergic transmitters are normally involved. Moreover, there is no monoamine oxidase in either human or cat glands. The dog's epitrichial glands respond to both adrenergic and cholinergic substances (Aoki, 1955), but it is doubtful whether these glands are normally under direct nervous control. The horse's glands can also be stimulated by both sorts of drugs, although they are probably normally controlled by circulating adrenaline and not by nervous stimulation (Evans and Smith, 1956). In sheep, goats (Robertshaw, 1968), pigs (Ingram, 1967), and donkeys (Robertshaw and Taylor, 1969) the glands respond to adrenergic but not cholinergic substances.

Denervation of the atrichial glands in man and the cat leads to loss of function and, after a period, to a loss of sensitivity toward drugs that normally stimulate them, and to the loss of cholinesterase. In the ox, unilateral sympathectomy abolishes the thermal response of the glands (Findlay and Robertshaw, 1965). However, in the horse, sweating breaks out within half an hour of the operation, probably because the consequent vasodilatation increases the blood supply to the glands. An intact nerve supply is not sufficient to ensure sweating in the ox, however, because if the blood supply to a limb is occluded the sweating response to a thermal stimulus is abolished (Ingram et al., 1963). Moreover, in man, arterial occlusion of a limb leads to a decrease in sweat production (Kuno, 1956).

Although both atrichial and epitrichial glands are loosely called sweat glands, their thermoregulatory significance varies among species and within species according to their location. Only a few species have been studied in any detail. Of these, man has received by far the most attention and so is considered separately.

Man

The glands on the palm of the hand and sole of the foot have no thermoregulatory function and, in fact, their secretion declines in the heat. The axillary glands may also respond to emotional stimuli and in any event contribute only a small proportion to the total evaporative loss.

On initial exposure to heat there is a variable delay of 5–40 minutes before sweating occurs, while body temperatures increase. The first signs of active sweating are detected on the lower part of the legs, beginning on the foot. With further increases in body temperature recruitment of sweat glands takes place on the abdomen, then the chest, and last on the head and forearm (Fig. 4–13) (Hertzman et al., 1952; Randall and Hertzman, 1953). At first the rate of water loss is low and Randall (1963) suggests that it is controlled at the spinal level. As the intensity of heating increases, however, there is within a given area an increase in the number of sweat glands that are active. Finally, an increased output by individual glands occurs. This pattern of sweating, beginning in the lower extremities, remains true even if only part of the body is heated. For example, in experiments in which only the upper part of the trunk is heated sweating still starts on the foot. In other words, sweating appears to be controlled by the overall demand for heat loss rather than by the temperature of the sweating surface, although local conditions near the glands are of importance (Ogawa, 1973).

During a period of sweating the output of a given area fluctuates and there are, similarly, variations in skin temperature. This has given rise to the idea that sweating may be controlled by variations in central rather than in peripheral temperatures. There are, however, a number of studies that point to a more complex control system, involving inputs from both the skin and the deep body thermosensors. The work of Benzinger (1959) and Benzinger et al. (1963), using a gradient layer calorimeter, is the chief source of evidence for those who support the idea that hypothalamic temperature is the most important factor in the control of sweating. Under the very carefully controlled conditions of these experiments, sweat rates were closely related to temperature changes

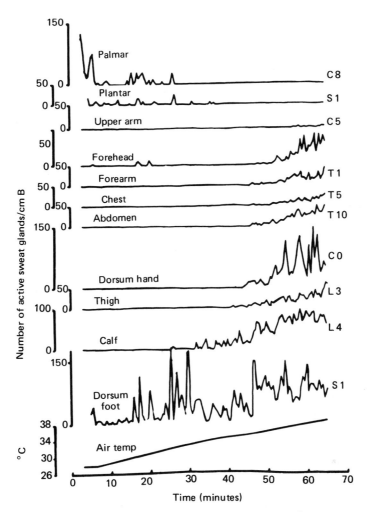

Fig. 4–13. The onset of sweating on various parts of the body in man on exposure to a rising ambient temperature (Randall and Hertzman, 1953).

on the tympanic membrane but not to changes in skin temperature. In spite of these studies, however, there are several other experiments that do not appear to fit in with Benzinger's hypothesis. For example, when the limbs are heated by immersing them in water while the blood supply is occluded, no change in deep body temperature occurs, although sweating is initiated (Randall, 1963).

Moreover, in other experiments it has been possible to show that cooling a small area of skin depresses sweating without there being a change in deep body temperature. This suggests an interaction of central and peripheral temperatures. During work in a hot climate sweating also appears to depend on both central and peripheral temperatures (Gisolfi and Robinson, 1970). Sweating may also occur below the lesion in the paraplegic man, although it is not as profuse as in the normal subject (Seckendorf and Randall, 1961). There is therefore little doubt that sweat rate can be influenced by changes in skin temperature without any change in hypothalamic temperatures, and sweating is probably controlled by the interaction of temperatures on the skin and deep in the body. Evidence in support of this idea has recently been provided, which suggests that the important variable is the mean body temperature (Snellen, 1967). This hypothesis can obviously explain sweating in a hot environment and during hard manual work (Wyndham et al., 1954) in a cool environment. The mechanism by which the local temperature of the skin influences the sweating rate probably involves an enhanced response of the gland to a constant nervous stimulus as temperature rises.

The actual amount of sweat produced by man depends on the severity of the heat load and on whether the subject is working. It also depends on sex, men producing more sweat than women (Fox et al., 1969; Wyndham et al., 1965). Over short periods of an hour, rates of over 4 liters/hour have been recorded under experimental conditions. Coal miners may have sweat rates of 2½ liters/hour and lose over 8 liters during a 5-hour working shift. In the desert, rates of water loss of 1½ liters/hour are common, and the total sweat loss may amount to 10–15 liters in the day (Schmidt-Nielsen, 1964). Reduction in water intake reduces water loss slightly, probably because body temperature increases during dehydration, so aiding heat loss. The saving, however, is only of the order of 10 percent. After man has been exposed to a hot climate, the amount of sweat produced increases because the glands increase their output; more glands do not become active (Collins and Weiner, 1962; Peter and Wyndham, 1966). Continuous prolonged exposure to severe heat, however, can result in the glands becoming fatigued and ceasing to function.

Schmidt-Nielsen (1964) has reviewed the problems of water replacement by sweating man and has shown that, in spite of the large amounts of water lost during exposure in the desert, man can do very little to prepare himself by drinking water before going out into the heat. Moreover, after the loss of even 10 liters of sweat, a man given free access to water becomes satisfied before the deficit is made up. Some further time must elapse before he can drink enough water to restore the balance completely (Chapters 9 and 10).

Other Mammals

The most famous of the desert mammals is the camel, and because of its ability to survive without water it has attracted the attention of those interested in water balance. Schmidt-Nielsen (1964) has studied this animal intensively and has found that although it sweats it does so with great economy. During the night, it allows its body temperature to fall and this, combined with its large bulk, enables it to store a considerable amount of heat during the day. Therefore, sweat production can be delayed while body temperature increases. This fluctuation in body temperature becomes even more marked during periods of dehydration, the body temperature falling to as low as 34°C and rising to nearly 41°C. In addition the sweat that is produced appears to evaporate on the skin rather than at the tip of the hairs, so the latent heat of vaporization is drawn from the skin rather than from the atmosphere.

A similar fluctuation in body temperature and a delay in the onset of sweating has also been reported in the donkey. In this species, however, body temperature does not increase to such a high value as in the camel before sweating begins. The donkey, in fact, is used widely under desert conditions and has been studied by Schmidt-Nielsen (1964), Bullard et al. (1970), and Robertshaw and Taylor (1969). They find that the animal is tolerant to dehydration and probably begins to sweat in response to both peripheral and central stimuli. Other large mammals, such as the eland, also display a capacity to reduce sweating by storing heat during the day (Taylor, 1970). The extent to which sweating can be delayed in these mammals depends on body size and the associated capacity to store heat.

McLean's (1963b) study of the ox has shown that European species dissipate 75 percent of their evaporative heat loss by sweating. The proportion is higher in *Bos indicus* because the contribution made by panting is lower. There is also evidence that breeds of cattle originating in the tropics have longer sweat glands (Pan, 1963) and evaporate more water from their body surface than temperate-zone breeds. As in other species, the control of the onset of sweating appears to depend partly on deep body temperature, because cattle sweat in response to warming of the hypothalamus (Ingram et al., 1963), and partly on peripheral stimulation.

In the sheep and goat, sweating is slight (Brook and Short, 1960) and intermittent and may stop after prolonged exposure (Robertshaw, 1968). In any event, when the glands discharge, the fleece takes up the moisture. Because of the heat released when wool is wetted, the skin temperature actually rises (Bligh, 1961). Apart from the function of the sweat glands on the scrotum (Waites and Voglmayr, 1963), therefore, the sweat glands in these species probably have little or no thermoregulatory significance.

The dog increases its water loss through the skin in response to local heating of the skin, but cutaneous vaporization of moisture is not an important avenue of heat loss in this species (Aoki and Wada, 1951). The pig does not sweat in the heat, although it possesses well-developed epitrichial glands (Ingram, 1964).

Behavioral Wetting of the Skin

Both panting and sweating involve the animal in the expenditure of some energy and may upset not only the water balance of the body but also the blood pCO_2 and the salt balance. Water applied to the outside of the body, however, provides a means of increasing evaporative heat loss without these

disadvantages. In some species, such as the water buffalo, which has practically no sweat glands, a wallow is essential for survival. Similarly, the heat tolerance of the pig can be greatly increased by the introduction of a mud wallow. Mud has some advantages over clean water simply because the cooling effect is prolonged by the water held in the mud. In an experiment on the pig, it has been found that in a warm environment a skin wetted with clean water produces an evaporation rate of 800 gm. m^{-2} hr^{-1} and is dry in about 15 minutes; when mud is used, the same high water loss is prolonged for nearly 2 hours (Ingram, 1965a).

The extent to which this form of cooling is effective depends partly on the nature of the skin. If the surface is covered with long dense hair, the water tends to be evaporated from the tips of the hair and much of the energy of vaporization is derived not from the animal but from the atmosphere. Such animals as the pig, hippopotamus, and elephant are therefore suited to such cooling, whereas the fully fleeced sheep is almost completely protected from water. Some small rodents, for example the rat, lick their fur under heat stress and so achieve a degree of evaporative cooling. This behavior is really only a last resort, however, and cannot be used over long periods as an effective method of thermoregulation.

In the absence of water, animals are known to wallow in urine or feces. The woodstork has developed a behavioral pattern under heat stress of excreting onto its legs, which are uninsulated and well vascularized (Kahl, 1963).

Effect of Humidity and the Capacity for Evaporative Heat Loss

It is obvious from personal experience that the degree of discomfort caused by high temperatures varies very much with the humidity. Such a correlation is to be expected, for the capacity of water to evaporate obviously depends on the degree of saturation of the air. For man, therefore, who is capable of such high rates of moisture vaporization, the wet bulb temperature is a better indicator of thermal comfort than the dry bulb temperature. In their study of heat stress and humidity on man, Provins et al. (1962) have found that the weighted temperature can best be expressed as:

Weighted temperature
$$= (WB \times 0.85) + (DB \times 0.15)$$

In cattle, which both sweat and pant but which nevertheless are not capable of such high rates of moisture vaporization, Bianca (1962) has found the following weighting satisfactory:

Weighted temperature
$$= (WB \times 0.65) + (DB \times 0.35)$$

In the pig, which does not sweat and is not very efficient at panting, the weighting for the wet bulb is even lower (Ingram, 1965b):

Weighted temperature
$$= (WB \times 0.35) + (DB \times 0.65)$$

The point of comparisons is that just as it is impossible to determine from the effects on one's own person whether another species is warm or cold in a given environment, or whether the air movement is causing an unacceptable heat loss, so it is also impossible to guess at the effects of humidity without knowing something about the animal's physiology.

Evaporative Heat Loss in Invertebrates

The problem associated with evaporative heat loss from terrestrial invertebrates have been reviewed by Cloudsley-Thompson (1970). Soft-skinned animals, such as earthworms and slugs, have no control over moisture loss and soon die from desiccation. Such animals seek shelter by burrowing or by selecting some damp microclimate under stones. Snails that have a shell and an operculum, however, may resist desiccation by withdrawing their bodies and sealing the entrance to the shell.

The problems of water balance in terrestrial arthropods has been extensively studied by Edney (1957). The outer, or epicuticle, layer of the bodies of many species is composed of a layer of wax that under most conditions is relatively impervious to water. Centipedes, millipedes, woodlice, and some arachnids and insects do lose water rapidly. During short exposures to high temperatures these animals may keep their body temperatures below the lethal limit, but because of their small body size they soon die from desiccation. Under the hot humid conditions of their microclimate, however, Edney has found that some woodlice are forced to come out into the sunlight where evaporation can occur; otherwise body temperature may reach the lethal limit. The amount of water lost in these circumstances depends entirely on the physical conditions and there is no evidence of control other than by the selection of microclimate.

Because the epicuticle of insects is waxy, some insects can display what appears to be a controlled evaporative loss. At high temperatures the cuticle "melts," becoming permeable to water (Wigglesworth, 1965), and an increased evaporative loss occurs. This tends to reduce temperature so that the wax solidifies again and the moisture loss is stopped. Cloudsley-Thompson (1970) points out, however, that this is hardly to be regarded as a physiological mechanism for controlling body temperature. In any event, death from desiccation is probably a greater danger than the threat of overheating in most instances.

Cooling in insects by a mechanism similar in some respects to panting has been demonstrated in the tsetse fly. In this species the spiracles on the thorax open rhythmically at temperatures above 30°C and open fully at 40°C, with the result that body temperature may be depressed by more than 1°C (Edney and Barass, 1962). Again, the capacity for evaporative cooling is very limited because of the small body size.

The bee exhibits a form of controlled evaporative heat loss of the hive, or more particularly of the developing larvae, by bringing in drops of moisture that are allowed to evaporate above the honeycomb cells. Generally speaking, however, controlled evaporative cooling, is not important in the invertebrates (Cloudsley-Thompson, 1970), as can be expected on general theoretical grounds for the same reasons that small mammals find it impracticable to employ the evaporation of moisture vapor for more than a short period.

CHAPTER 5

The Cardiovascular System

Although the temperature of the body core in mammals and birds is maintained at a fairly constant level, the temperature of the peripheral tissue may vary widely. The effect of these variations in temperature, which are usually associated with changes in the thickness of the peripheral shell, is to modify the resistance to heat loss (Chapter 2). In animals with an external insulation in the form of feathers or fur, the resistance to heat flow can be increased in the cold by piloerection, or "fluffing up" the coat, with the result that the amount of trapped air is increased. In man a similar effect is obtained when he wears extra clothes. Within the peripheral tissue, heat conductance is modified by variations in the flow rate of blood that transfers heat from deep in the core to the skin surface. Even under thermoneutral conditions, however, external insulation is already near its minimum. On exposure to heat, therefore, an increased peripheral blood flow plays an important role in increasing the rate of heat loss. In animals that sweat, and particularly in man with his very high rate of cutaneous moisture loss, the increased blood flow provides both the latent heat of vaporization and a supply of water for evaporation.

The capacity for a given surface to lose heat depends partly on its position and partly on the degree of external insulation. In many animals, the external insulation on the extremities is not as thick as that on the trunk and this enhances their value as radiators. In addition, the extremities have a high surface area to volume ratio and may be exposed to air currents that have not been conditioned by passing over other parts of the body. Even the surface of the trunk itself may take on some of these features as, for example, the folds of skin (dewlap) that hang down from the neck and abdomen of tropical cattle. A part of the body that is exposed directly to the sun, however, may actually experience a net gain of heat from the environment and a high rate of blood flow is therefore instrumental in transfering heat into the body core. Under these conditions, much depends on the rate of cutaneous moisture loss in determining whether the increased rate of blood flow actually helps to dissipate heat. There is, however, some evidence to support the idea that when the radiant heat load is high and the surface temperature is above 40°C blood flow decreases again and so limits the passage of heat into the core.

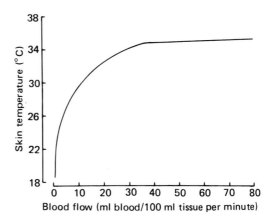

Fig. 5–1. Relation between blood flow in the finger and skin temperature (redrawn from Aschoff and Wever, 1957).

Effects of Environmental Temperature on Peripheral Blood Flow in Man

Accounts of the various methods for measuring blood flow through the peripheral tissue are available in reviews by Greenfield (1963) and Thauer (1965). The methods are of significance because to some extent they have set limits on the possible types of experiments. All the techniques have their particular advantages and disadvantages and it is important that these be appreciated when the results of a given study are evaluated. Special care must be taken in the use of indirect methods.

Skin temperature, for example, is a relatively easy measurement to take. Although it can be used to indicate changes in blood flow, however, its usefulness is limited to a particular range of skin temperatures and, of course, changes in ambient temperature must be taken into account. The relations between some of these measurements are illustrated in the studies by Aschoff and Wever (1957) and Burton and Edholm (1955), who have recorded several variables simultaneously. In Fig. 5–1 it can be seen that an increase in blood flow in the finger, as measured directly by venous occlusion plethysmography, is accompanied by large changes in skin temperature. However, whereas a change in blood flow from 0 to 10 ml/per 100 ml tissue per minute is associated with a 16°C change in skin temperature, further increases in blood flow up to 80 ml per 100 ml tissue per

minute cause hardly any temperature change at all.

In contrast, measurements of thermal conductivity, that is, heat flow per unit length in unit time (Fig. 5–2), have a close rela-

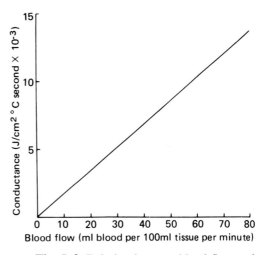

Fig. 5–2. Relation between blood flow and conductance in the finger (redrawn from Aschoff and Wever, 1957).

tion to blood flow over a wide range. Although several methods are based on conductivity measurements, there are nevertheless limitations, discussed by Thauer (1965), that relate chiefly to keeping the conditions constant while measurements are made. Conductance (heat loss per unit area per degree temperature gradient in unit time) also displays a close correlation with blood flow but, again, it is only applicable under steady-state conditions.

A common feature of methods for measuring peripheral blood flow quantitatively is that they are best suited for use on a cooperative subject who is not moving about. Consequently, the greater part of our knowledge is derived from studies on man. Blood flow in the arm, hand, or finger can be estimated directly from the increase in volume of the extremity when the venous return is prevented (venous occlusion plethysmography). Basically, the method involves placing the extremity (finger, hand, arm, leg) into a closed compartment that is filled with either air or water. The venous return from the extremity is then occluded by the inflation of a cuff to diastolic pressure and hence for a short time blood flows into the limb but not out. During this period the increase in volume of the limb in unit time is measured and because this additional volume is all blood, the rate of flow can be expressed in terms of milliliters of blood per 100 ml tissue per minute.

The interpretation of measurements, however, is complicated by the fact that at plethysmograph temperatures between 33 °C and 43 °C blood flow is variable even when the temperature conditions are kept constant. At first, after an increase in ambient temperature, there is an increase in flow rate. After an hour or so it declines, for reasons that are not fully understood but the effects of which nevertheless must be taken into account. That the increased blood flow in a limb is in the skin rather than in the muscle has been established in a number of studies, such as that by Edholm et al. (1956). In this study the flow of blood in the skin has been stopped by iontophoresis of adrenaline, while total blood flow rate is measured. In fact, muscle blood flow tends to decline when total blood flow in a limb increases in response to heat.

In experiments involving the use of a water plethysmograph two variables are under the experimenter's direct control. One is the ambient temperature of the room, and the other is the temperature of the vessel containing the extremity. Both have proved to be of importance in the regulation of blood flow in a limb. At a constant ambient temperature in the room, blood flow depends on the temperature of the water in the plethysmograph, higher temperatures being associated with a high blood flow, as happens when the hands are washed in hot water. The changes in blood flow are almost linearly related to the temperature of the plethysmograph above about 22 °C, although the slope of the line does become steeper at higher environmental temperatures. When the plethysmograph temperature is kept constant, blood flow increases as the environmental temperature increases. Under these conditions, at air temperatures above 28 °C, the increase in blood flow with air temperature is again almost linear, except that the slope of the line becomes steeper at high plethysmograph temperatures (Fig. 5–3). Results of this kind suggest that local blood flow can be influenced both by local thermal stimuli and by stimuli applied elsewhere on the body.

This was demonstrated many times in other types of experiments, which usually involved placing one limb in warm water and measuring blood flow in another limb (Lewis and Pickering, 1931; Gibbons and Landis, 1932; Pickering and Hess, 1933). In these early experiments, there was a gain of heat by the blood circulating through the limb that was immersed in warm water and vasodilatation in unheated extremities did not occur until 10 minutes or more after heating began. It therefore appeared that the increased blood flow in the unheated extremities could be related to a rise in deep body temperature. Other types of study, in which the consumption of hot drinks was followed by vasodilatation, supported the idea that central receptors were important. Moreover, it was also shown that the injection of

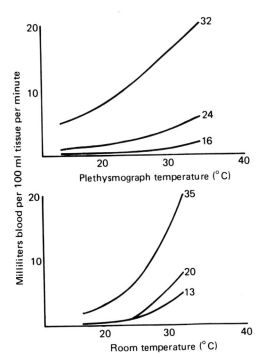

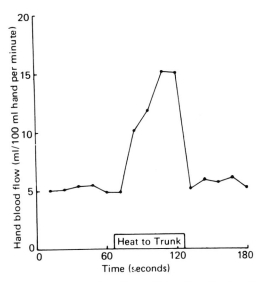

Fig. 5–4. The effect of heating the trunk on blood flow in the hand (from Cooper and Kerslake, 1954).

Fig. 5–3. In the upper graph blood flow has been plotted against the temperature of the water in the plethysmograph for different room temperatures of 16°C, 24°C, and 32°C. In the lower graph the same data have been plotted as blood flow against room temperature for plethysmograph temperatures of 13°C, 20°C, and 35°C (drawn from the data of Spealman, 1945).

warm saline into the blood stream could cause vasodilatation (Snell, 1954).

Later studies, however, have reinforced the importance of peripheral nervous pathways in the control of blood flow. The results displayed in Fig. 5–4 relate to the effect of heating the trunk with an infrared lamp on blood flow in the hand (Cooper and Kerslake, 1954). It can be seen that vasodilatation occurs with almost no delay and is accompanied by a slight fall in core temperature. In order to investigate the problem further Cooper and Kerslake (1954) have carried out tests in which the legs are exposed to infrared heat only as far as the midthigh. Heating the legs is then followed by vasodilatation in the hand, even when the venous return from the leg is prevented by

a cuff inflated to a pressure of 250 mm Hg. In control experiments it has been shown that inflation of the cuff alone does not affect the circulation in the hand. These results clearly demonstrate the role of a nervous pathway in the control of reflex vasodilatation. They are supported by studies on patients with unilateral sympathectomy (Fig. 5–5) in which heating the sympathectomized leg fails to cause vasodilatation elsewhere. Reflex vasodilatation nevertheless depends

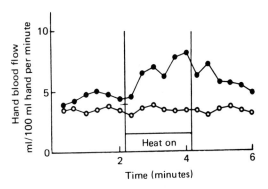

Fig. 5–5. The effect on blood flow in the hand of heating a normal leg (●—●) and a sympathectomized leg (○—○) (Cooper and Kerslake, 1954).

on ambient temperature because it does not occur in a cold environment.

As already mentioned, changes in the temperature of the body core are also important in the control of peripheral blood flow; in a hot environment, when body temperature is liable to increase, its effect must be taken into account. Experiments involving the local heating or cooling of structures deep in the body are limited to animals, but changes in body temperature measured on the eardrum have been recorded by Benzinger (1959, 1969) from humans in a gradient layer calorimeter. In these studies, blood flow has been estimated indirectly from changes in the conductance of the whole body and plotted against skin temperature, on the one hand, and eardrum temperature, on the other. The results demonstrate not only the effect of peripheral temperature on conductance but also a strong influence of core temperature.

Under hot ambient conditions, the difference between skin temperature and the surroundings is much reduced and, as a consequence, so is the capacity to lose heat by convection and radiation. Much more important is the evaporation of water. In man, with his high sweat rates, therefore, it is perhaps not surprising that evidence has been found that the sweat glands are responsible for producing a substance called "bradykinin," which is a powerful vasodilator (Fox and Hilton, 1958; Fox et al., 1961). Part, at least, of the high peripheral blood flow in man in a hot environment may then be related to the local effects of sweating. This factor adds a further complication to the problem of the nervous control of peripheral blood flow, a subject that has been reviewed by Hertzman (1959). It appears that there are two mechanisms involved:

1. A vasoconstrictor mediated by sympathetic nerves. Stimulation of these nerves, or the injection of noradrenaline, leads to vasoconstriction, whereas the release of the constrictor tone, as after sympa-

thectomy, leads, at least initially, to vasodilatation.

2. An "active" vasodilator that is mediated through sympathetic cholinergic fibres.

These conclusions are drawn from experiments in which blood flow through two similar areas is compared while one of the areas is denervated. From experiments of this kind it is apparent that not all parts of the body's periphery behave in the same way. In the hand and foot, and also in the ear and nose, the increase in blood flow on exposure to heat can be accounted for almost entirely by the release of vasoconstrictor tone. If the nerve supply is blocked, the skin vasodilates even in a cool environment, and there is no further increase in flow on exposure to heat. In the arms and legs, in contrast, there is almost no constrictor tone in the skin vessels, even at neutral ambient temperatures. If the nerve supply to the skin is blocked with atropine in one arm and the subject is exposed to heat, blood flow in that arm remains almost constant, whereas flow rate in the control arm increases considerably. The slight increase in flow in the blocked arm on initial exposure to heat suggests that there may be a further release of constrictor tone. The large increase in blood flow in the control arm, however, is related to an active vasodilatation mediated through nerves which release acetylcholine, for it does not occur after the nerve is blocked with atropine. This active vasodilatation is believed to be mediated indirectly by the release of bradykinin from the sweat glands, which have been stimulated through the sudomotor nerves. The observation that in the forearm the increased blood flow occurs at the same time or a little after sweating begins supports these ideas.

It should nevertheless be pointed out that this cannot be the complete story, because the sweat glands on the hand produce bradykinin, although there is no sign of active vasodilatation. In some experiments (Hertzman, 1959), moreover, there appears to be no close correlation between sweating and increased blood flow. In addition, some regions of the body, for example, the forehead, appear to have no vasoconstrictor tone, although there is active vasodilatation in the heat.

In the foregoing discussion almost all measurements of blood flow have been made in limbs. Blood flow on the trunk cannot readily be measured directly and must therefore be estimated from total body conductance. From studies by a number of workers it is evident that the range of blood flow changes over the trunk is much smaller than that in the limbs (between 1:3 and 1:6 according to Thauer, 1965). Moreover, the evidence from total body conductances suggests that although limb blood flow does not reach a minimum until about 20°C, blood flow in the trunk is steady below 28°C in man. Thauer (1965), however, states that there are limitations to the extent to which measurements of conductance can be used as quantitative measurements of blood flow and holds the view that blood flow on the trunk continues to decline below an ambient temperature of 28°C.

Effects of Environmental Temperature on Peripheral Blood Flow in Animals Other than Man

Because of the difficulties of using established techniques for quantitively estimating blood flow on animals, greater use has been made of temperature measurements of the skin and, where quantitative estimations have been made, the animal has sometimes been anesthetized. The anesthetic itself may influence blood flow and for this reason the observations made in some studies are of only limited significance. However, it has been possible to investigate the role of local

changes in deep body temperature much more fully in animals than in man by the use of implanted thermodes.

Mammals

Studies on a number of different animals suggest that blood flow in the extremities is controlled by several variables just as in man, but there are some differences among species. For example, in sheep, pigs, cattle, dogs, and rabbits, the temperature on the pinna of the ear changes abruptly as environmental temperature rises, indicating a sudden increase in blood flow associated with the opening of arteriovenous anastomoses. By contrast, Grant (1963) was unable to detect similar changes in the temperature of the rat's ear, which has no arteriovenous anastomoses, although sudden changes in temperature were detected in the feet and tail. These differences are in fact related to the absence of arteriovenous anastomoses in the rat because there is known to be a sympathetic nerve supply in the rat's ear. There is a major difference between man and many other mammals, in so far as in the latter, the increase in blood flow through the extremities can with certain exceptions (e.g., the muskrat) be accounted for by the release of vasoconstrictor tone (Green et al., 1956). Possibly an active vasodilatation does not have a selective advantage in evolution for most species until the efficiency of the sweat glands is improved to the point seen in man. Even those lower mammals that sweat do so at a rate much lower than man. Therefore, a high rate of blood flow that takes large quantities of heat and water to the body surface is not of any great advantage to the animal.

A consequence of blood flow being controlled by release of constrictor tone, of course, is that if most of the tone is lost on initial exposure to heat then there is little further increase at very high ambient temperatures. Whittow (1962) has judged from measurements of skin temperature in the ox that peripheral blood flow may be of limited importance in increasing sensible heat loss in a very warm environment. Once the tissue insulation has been reduced to a certain value the resistance to heat loss lies principally in the external insulation, provided by the coat, which remains constant. On the other hand as the ox is a sweating animal, the role of the blood supply to the sweat glands should not be overlooked.

The role of blood flow through the extremities in rodents has been considered by Hart (1971). In these animals the tail is of particular importance and, as in man, there is some indication that blood flow changes occur in the extremities at lower environmental temperatures than on the trunk. Rand et al. (1965) have measured blood flow

through the tail of the rat by means of venous occlusion plethysmography at various ambient temperatures. They have found that flow rate increases considerably at about the critical temperature of 28°C and as much as 20 per cent of the heat loss at high temperatures is through the tail (Fig. 5–6). However, the relation of flow rate to temperature is considerably influenced by the previous thermal history of the animals. The muskrat (Johansen, 1962) also uses its tail to dissipate heat, and blood flow as measured by venous occlusion plethysmography has been shown to vary with the temperature of the water in which the tail is immersed. Blockage of the nerves to the muskrat's tail with local anesthetic prevents vasodilatation there in a hot environment and body temperature rises. In the muskrat, therefore, there appears to be an active vasodilatation, although the mechanism is not

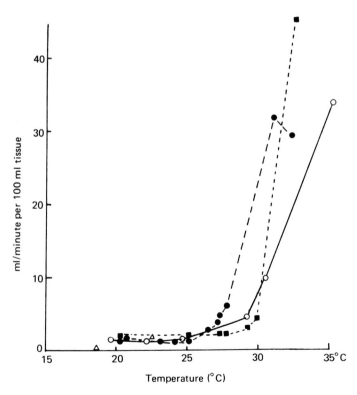

Fig. 5–6. Blood flow in the tail of the rat at different environmental temperatures (based on the data of Rand et al., 1965; reproduced by permission of the National Research Council of Canada).

known. When the muskrat tail is vasodilated, injection of adrenaline is followed immediately by vasoconstriction. The importance of the tail in the beaver has been demonstrated by Steen and Steen (1965), who have shown that when the naturally naked tail is placed in cold water an air temperature of up to 25°C can be tolerated, although when the whole animal is exposed to air above 20°C it becomes hyperthermic.

Increases in temperature on the surface of the dog's ear and on the paws of cats and dogs have been shown to occur on exposure to a hot ambient. The extent to which these regions can contribute to heat loss, however, is limited by the insulation of the fur. The foot pad, which is naked, can provide a site of heat loss but only, of course, when it is in contact with a cool surface.

In cattle, Whittow (1962) and Ingram and Whittow (1962a,b,c) have shown that large increases in the temperature of the shank may occur (1) on exposure to a high temperature; (2) when body temperature increases after eating (Fig. 5–7); and (3)

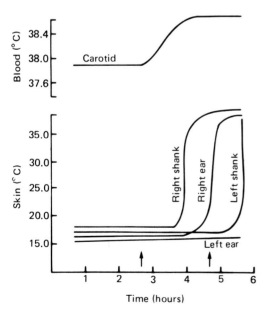

Fig. 5–7. The effect of feeding on skin temperatures on the ears and the shanks of the leg of the ox (redrawn from Ingram and Whittow, 1962b).

when the trunk is exposed to infrared heat. In the latter instance, the ears and forelimbs have been shaded from the radiant heat lamps in order to eliminate direct effects. In some instances, extremity temperatures increase after a delay of up to 2 hours, when body temperature has also increased, but in other cases the increase is almost immediate and involves no change in the temperature of the blood in the carotid artery.

Similar increases in the temperature of the extremities have been observed in sheep. Blaxter et al. (1959) have published data demonstrating that under some conditions heat loss from the sparsely covered parts of the sheep may account for a considerable part of the total heat loss. The horns of artiodactyls are also subject to temperature changes associated with variations in blood flow. Taylor (1966) has measured heat loss from the goat's horn but doubts whether it is of importance in a hot climate. He points out, however, that some species wallow with their horns, and for these the heat loss may be of no little significance.

Measurements of blood flow on the trunk of conscious animals by direct methods is difficult, as it is in man, but inferences can be drawn from changes in tissue insulation and the thermal circulation index. In the young pig (Ingram, 1964b), tissue insulation falls abruptly between 25°C and 30°C ambient temperature. The thermal circulation index also changes at the same time as the temperature of the ear increases from just above ambient temperature to near 35°C. These results are similar to those obtained for man (Burton and Edholm, 1955) and for the sheep that has been clipped of its wool (Blaxter et al., 1959) and suggest that the changes in blood flow through the skin of the trunk are of comparable magnitude in all three species when exposed to a hot environment.

Studies involving the use of thermodes implanted within the hypothalamus have demonstrated that local changes of temperature in this region are accompanied by changes in blood flow through the extremities. In the anesthetized cat, blood flow through the limbs, as measured directly by collecting the outflow, increases in response to warming the hypothalamus, and the increase is greater at high ambient temperatures (Ström, 1950). Similarly, it has been demonstrated in the conscious cat, dog, goat, pig, and ox that warming the hypothalamus increases blood flow in the skin. The effect is more pronounced in a warm environment than in a cold one. Conversely, cooling the hypothalamus tends to decrease peripheral blood flow (Fig. 5–8).

Another region of the nervous system where local temperature changes influence peripheral blood flow, as well as other temperature-regulating systems, is the spinal cord (Thauer, 1970; Simon, 1968). Warming of the spinal cord is accompanied by vasodilatation in the extremities, and cooling tends to cause vasoconstriction. Moreover, cooling the hypothalamus while the spine is being heated reduces the extent of the vasodilatation. Part, at least, of the influence of the neurones in the spine that regulate peripheral blood flow appears to be independent of the hypothalamus, because adjustments to

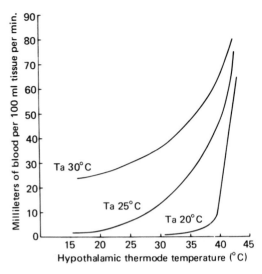

Fig. 5–8. The effect of changing the temperature of a thermode in the hypothalamus on blood flow in the tail of a pig at environmental temperatures (Ta) of 20°C, 25°C, and 30°C (based on the data of Ingram and Legge, 1971).

blood flow are still seen in response to changes in the temperature of the spinal cord in the chronically spinalized dog (Walther et al., 1971) (Fig. 5–9).

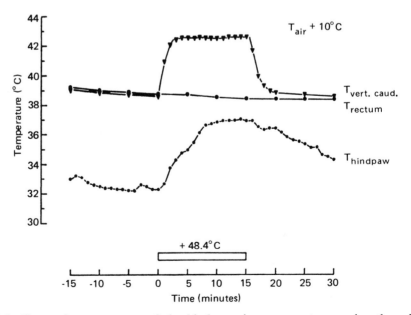

Fig. 5–9. Change in temperature of the hind paw in response to warming the spinal cord (bar) in a dog 19 days after spinal transection (Walther et al., 1971).

Vasomotor changes that occur in response to ambient temperature are thus controlled by a complex of signals. An attempt to investigate how these are integrated has been made in the pig (Ingram and Legge, 1971). In these studies, blood flow has been measured in the tails of conscious animals by means of venous occlusion plethysmography. The temperature on the skin of the trunk has been controlled independently of the environmental temperature by means of a coat through which water can be circulated. Ambient temperature around the head and extremities is controlled by the air temperature of the room and thermodes are placed along the spine and in the hypothalamus. These studies have demonstrated that blood flow is influenced by (1) the temperature of the ambient air, (2) the temperature on the skin of the trunk, (3) the temperature of the spinal cord, (4) the temperature of the hypothalamus, and (5) the local effect of air movement round the tail (Fig. 5–10). Each factor appears to extend its influence independently of the others and the simplest explanation is that all the signals are fed into a central integrating system, which then determines the response. The result is that in a warm environment, when skin temperature is high and body temperature is slightly elevated, cooling the spine or the hypothalamus or even both together does not cause complete vasoconstriction. In a cool environment, heating thermodes in the core may not cause vasodilatation. In the intact animal, the autonomous regulation that can be demonstrated in isolated systems appears to be largely overridden.

Birds

The feathers provide a thick layer of insulation over the trunk and beneath them the temperature of the skin alters very little over a wide range of ambient temperatures. The legs, comb, and wattle, however, which have no external insulation, increase their surface temperature considerably when the ambient temperature increases, as illustrated by the work of Wilson et al. (1952) (Fig. 5–11). Heating the body trunk, but not the extremities, also leads to increases in temperature of the uninsulated surfaces. The large changes in skin temperature must be the result of changes in blood flow. They enable the bird to lose excess heat, particularly from the legs, which to some extent are shaded from the sun and in some species may be immersed in water.

Information about various species of birds has been collected by Dawson and Hudson (1970). They demonstrate that thermal conductance increases by a factor of between two and three when ambient temperature rises from 20°C to 40°C, and this implies an increase in peripheral blood flow. The body temperature of birds tends to be higher than in mammals. With a moderate degree of hyperthermia, a significant portion of the heat production may still be lost by

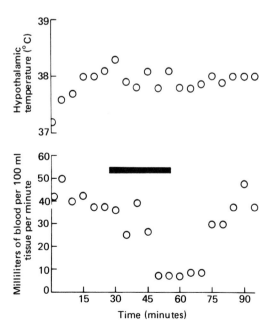

Fig. 5–10. Effect of increase in air movement (black bar) on blood flow in the pig's tail (from Ingram and Legge, 1971).

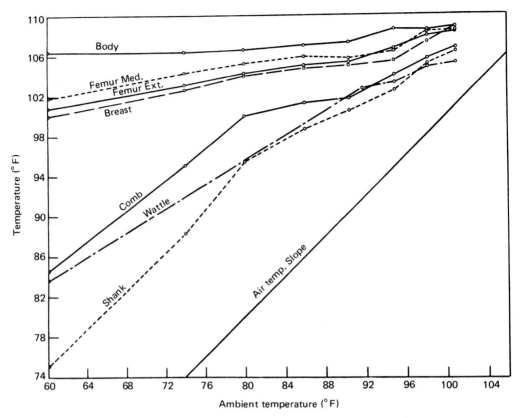

Fig. 5–11. Relation between ambient temperature and body surface temperatures in the hen. The air temperature slope represents the isotherm between skin and air temperature (Wilson et al., 1952).

nonevaporative channels, even in an ambient temperature of 40°C. Although birds have not received as much attention as mammals, it therefore appears that a similar pattern of blood-flow changes occurs in the heat.

Reptiles

Exposure to hot environments in lizards has a marked effect on the cardiovascular system in general because heart rate, cardiac output, and blood pressure all increase as body temperature rises. Templeton (1970) has reviewed the problem and has pointed out that, although arterial pressure increases

as the core temperature rises, it reaches a fairly constant value above 25°C in spite of a continued increase in cardiac output. The peripheral resistance must therefore change, although the vasodilatation that controls this resistance need not be confined to the skin. Evidence indicating that the circulation to the skin is specifically involved, however, derives from the studies of Bartholomew and Tucker (1963). They have heated and cooled both living and dead lizards and have recorded the changes in body temperature. Living animals change core temperature more quickly (as is to be expected) because the circulation distributes heat about the body. In contrast to dead animals, however, the living ones heat up more rapidly than they cool down (Fig. 5–12).

Blood Flow and Heat Loss

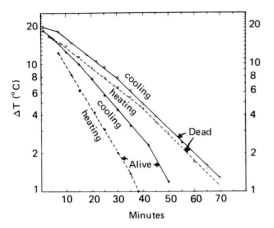

Fig. 5–12. Effects of heating by exposure to air at 40°C and cooling by exposure to air at 20°C on a lizard while it is alive, and after it is dead. ΔT is the difference between air temperature and body temperature (Bartholomew and Tucker, 1963; copyright University of Chicago).

The extent to which changes in blood flow rate can be related to changes in heat loss has been examined by Thauer (1965). From his account, it is clear that a direct relation between blood flow and heat loss is established over only a very limited range of conditions. Heat loss through the tissue of the skin is proportional to tissue conductance times the difference between core and skin temperature:

$$H = k(T_c - T_s)$$

Even if tissue conductance and blood flow are regarded as exactly interchangeable quantities, heat loss is proportional to blood flow only as long as $(T_c - T_s)$ remains constant. In a hot environment, the temperature of the body core tends to rise and the change in skin temperature depends on core temperature and environmental temperature as well as on the extent to which moisture is evaporated from the surface. This last term, in turn, depends on the amount of sweating and on the humidity of the ambient air.

For a given body temperature, heart rate is higher during heating than during cooling, suggesting differences in the circulation of the blood. Measurement of the thermal conductance of lizards reveals that it is greater during heating, which indicates that the animal vasodilates and consequently gains heat rapidly, whereas vasoconstriction in a cool environment reduces the rate at which the body temperature falls. These findings extend and confirm those of Cowles (1958), who has demonstrated that the temperature gradient across the skin of the desert iguana is smaller while the animal is being heated than while it is being cooled. This investigator suggests that the control of dermal blood flow has been developed in amphibia in connection with the respiratory function of the skin; has been modified in reptiles, in which it serves to prolong the period of activity by increasing the rate of warming and decreasing the rate of cooling; and finally has developed in the birds and mammals as a true thermoregulatory mechanism.

Blood flow changes are greater in the extremities than on the trunk and immersion of a limb into hot water results in a gain in heat when water temperature rises above core temperature. In spite of this gain of heat, further heating of the water results in an even greater blood flow, which conducts heat even faster into the core. One advantage of this conduction of heat away from the surface is that local skin temperature tends to be protected from an excessive rise in temperature. Exposure to high air temperatures can also result in very high blood flows. Because sweating also occurs, however, the high flow rates serve to transport heat and water to the sweat glands and there is a net loss of heat. Under conditions of very high humidity, when heat loss by sweating is limited, heat is again transferred into the body just as when the limb is immersed in water.

The point that emerges from these considerations is that before heat loss and blood flow are equated with each other, the environmental and physiological conditions must be examined very carefully.

Special Arrangements of Blood Vessels that Influence the Transfer of Heat

The transfer of heat to regions of the body where it can be lost to the environment and the protection of certain regions from excessive changes in temperature are influenced by the anatomical arrangement of blood vessels. The testes, for example, must be maintained at a temperature that is below core temperature in mammals (see Chapter 6) and yet must also be supplied with arterial blood. Both these conditions are met by a special arrangement of blood vessels in which the arterial and venous vessels are divided into small branches and closely applied to each other, over a long tortuous route, in a structure called the "pampiniform plexus." The cool venous blood thus removes heat from the arterial blood supply on its way through the plexus, which acts as a countercurrent heat exchanger.

A similar heat exchange function has been suggested for the carotid rete. In some species, the blood supply to the hypothalamus runs via a rete of arterial vessels, which consists of a system of branching and joining tubes that were compared by Galen to a fisherman's net (Fig. 5–13). This rete lies within a venous sinus that receives blood from the nasal passage, where it has been cooled. The arterial blood on its way to the brain thus passes through a heat exchanger and the hypothalamus is protected from an excessively high temperature. Animals that have a carotid rete may therefore be able to survive tem-

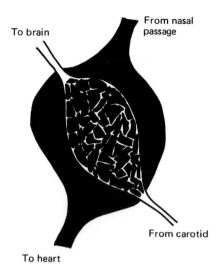

Fig. 5–13. Diagram of the carotid rete and the venous sinus within which it lies.

peratures in the body core that would be injurious to the brain.

Heat exchangers have been described in various situations (see review by Schmidt-Nielsen, 1963) and are well developed in the appendages of whales and the sloth (Scholander and Krog, 1957) but the emphasis that has been laid on them is in the protection of the body against heat loss in the cold. Arrangements that limit the loss of heat, however, are liable to prove a disadvantage if the animal is exposed to a hot environment and it is found that provision exists for the heat exchanger to be switched off in such an event.

In man, for example, the arterial supply of the arm is accompanied by two veins that are closely applied to it so that in a cold ambient, heat exchange takes place between the cool venous blood and the warm arterial supply. The result is that instead of heat being lost to the environment it can be returned to the core. In addition, there is an alternative venous drainage to the arm that runs via vessels close to the surface (Fig. 5–14). In a hot environment, blood is diverted from the veins close to the artery to the surface veins, where it continues to lose heat as it returns to the core. For example,

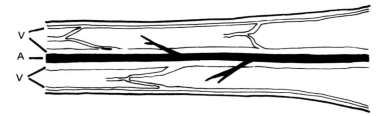

Fig. 5–14. Diagram of blood vessels in the arm. Blood may return by the surface veins (V) and bypass the heat exchanger, or blood may return via the veins close to the artery (A) where heat exchange can take place.

Bazett (1949) has found that in man in a warm environment venous blood is 35.1°C at the tip of the finger and only 34.6°C at the elbow. In a cool environment the gradient is reversed. The mechanism controlling the change in the path of the venous return has been investigated by Webb-Peploe and Shepherd (1969) in the dog. It depends on both local peripheral temperature and deep body temperature.

Within the skin surface the arrangement of the small blood vessels is similar in a wide range of mammals and consists of three interconnected plexuses lying within the dermis. The first plexus lies at the base of the dermis, just above the fat layer, and is made up of relatively large vessels that communicate with the plexus above and the deeper blood vessels (Fig. 5–15). Within the plexus, arteries and veins branch and join freely, forming a fine network of vessels. An arterial vessel is frequently accompanied by two veins lying close to it, although some arteries and veins run separately. Such an arrangement of small veins and arteries lying close together may be seen in many organs throughout the body and in all instances represents a countercurrent heat exchanger. In the skin, this tends to limit the transfer of heat to the surface. The presence of other arteries and veins, however, which are separate from each other, raises at least the possibility that the heat exchanger may be cut off in a warm environment. The second plexus is similar to the first but is made up of smaller vessels and lies between the sebaceous glands and the sweat glands. In some

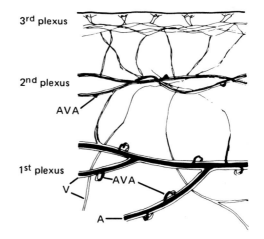

Fig. 5–15. Diagram of blood vessels in the skin. The vessels lie in three plexuses, the third being nearest to the surface. The arteriovenous anastomosis (AVA) allows blood to pass from an arterial vessel (A) to a venous vessel (V) without first going through the capillaries.

species, for example, sheep and pig, this plexus is poorly represented and consists in part of vessels that run horizontally for a short distance in passing between the first and the third plexus. The third plexus lies just beneath the epidermis and consists of small vessels that supply and drain the capillaries.

The flow of blood within the skin depends partly on whether the arterioles are open and allow blood to pass through the capillaries and partly on whether the arteriovenous anastomoses (AVAs) are open or closed. The AVAs are short vessels with muscular walls that join an artery to a vein.

When they are open, blood short circuits the route through the capillaries and returns to the heart. These structures are seen in the skin, particularly in the ears and extremities, but have also been observed in the skin covering the trunk of some species. They occur mainly in the first plexus but may also be seen at the level of the second. They are innervated by sympathetic nerves.

When the AVAs in the ear open, the flow of blood increases considerably. A similar situation probably occurs in the skin. The exact route taken by the blood is not clear, however. Under cold conditions the periodic warming of the extremities by the passage of blood depends on the AVAs opening, but if the arterioles remain closed, all the blood flow is short circuited. In a hot ambient, in contrast, both the AVAs and the arterioles may be open together. In this instance, the resistance to blood flow is not only lower, but blood and therefore heat can be taken closer to the surface. The extent to which blood flows through the alternative routes in the skin and the effect on heat loss is not completely understood, but the anatomical arrangement of the vessels clearly allows a number of possibilities.

The important lesson to be drawn from a study of the anatomy of the blood vessels is that, because of the countercurrent heat exchanger and the arteriovenous anastomoses, increases in blood flow may not necessarily be associated with an increase in the rate of heat flow of the magnitude expected. Even when a heat exchanger is not bypassed on exposure to a hot environment, an increased rate of blood flow reduces its efficiency simply because less time is available for heat to be exchanged.

Change in Vasomotor Tone of Resistance and Capacity Vessels

Peripheral resistance to blood flow is determined mostly by the proportion of arterioles that are constricted, whereas the effective capacity of the blood system depends on the vasomotor tone in the veins. The changes in blood flow that occur in response to changes in ambient temperature involve chiefly the resistance vessels, but the larger, capacity vessels may also make a contribution. Moreover, the changes in vasomotor tone in the resistance and capacity vessels may on occasion be out of phase. For example, after exposure to cold the small resistance vessels of a limb dilate soon after warming has begun, but the venous resistance may remain high for some time. At temperatures above the thermoneutral zone, however, the muscular tone in the walls of the veins is already low and the possible further increase in distensibility with increase in temperature is small. The contribution of changes in the capacity vessels to blood flow in a warm environment is therefore also small.

Changes in Blood Flow with Changes in Posture

Except in very severe heat exposure, changes in blood flow that are related to changes in blood pressure are small. Pressure changes that are related to posture can be significant, however. When the arm is raised above the head, arterial pressure in the fingers is effectively reduced by an amount equal to the height of the hand above the heart. In a cool environment, when blood flow in the hand is only moderate, the decrease in perfusion pressure caused by raising the hand can readily be offset by vasodilatation, which reduces the resistance. The result is that blood flow is only slightly reduced. Under hot conditions, the blood vessels in the hand are already dilated and there is a high rate of blood flow. Consequently, if the arm is raised above the head there can be no further vasodilatation to reduce peripheral resistance and so compensate for the reduction in transmural pressure. The result is that in a warm environment, when the hand is raised, blood flow falls considerably and reaches about the same low level as that observed when the hand is raised in a cool environment.

Another consequence of vasodilatation in a warm environment in relation to posture is the increased tendency to fainting and dizzyness. In the upright position and in the absence of muscle movement, blood tends to pool in the lower limbs and the decreased venous return may limit the cardiac output and cause fainting. When the ambient temperature is high both the resistance and the capacity vessels are dilated in the legs. The tendency for blood to pool and the subject to faint is therefore increased. These effects can best be demonstrated on the tilt table, where the subject can be changed passively from a supine to an erect position. In such a maneuver, there is always a tendency to faint but this is much greater in a hot ambient. Under these conditions the capacity vessels are dilated. In the supine position, venous pressure is so low that the vessels collapse; in cross section they are dumbbell shaped, with only narrow open pathways. On return to the erect position, the vessels fill. While this happens, venous return to the heart is very much reduced. The consequence is that the subject nearly always faints, although after acclimatization the incidence of syncope is reduced.

Compensatory Changes in Vascular Beds

The network of tubes making up the vascular system has a capacity that is greater than the volume of circulating blood. It follows that complete vasodilatation would result in circulatory collapse, as in shock. If the peripheral resistance were to remain constant at all times it would be necessary for the vasodilatation of one vascular bed to be balanced by vasoconstriction in another. In fact, peripheral resistance does not remain constant but there is evidence that vasodilatation of the skin in the heat is accompanied by some reduction in blood flow in other parts. The kidney, for example, may undergo a considerable reduction in blood flow. Under conditions of exercise in the heat, flow may be as low as 50 percent of the control value (Smith et al., 1952). The splanchnic blood supply is believed to be reduced generally on exposure to heat (Grayson, 1949), although few observations have been made and some of the reports are conflicting. Local heating of the spinal cord that results in an increased blood flow to the skin has been shown by direct measurements to be accompanied by a fall in blood flow to the intestine (Kullman et al., 1970). Muscle blood flow, as mentioned above, changes very little on heat exposure, although there is a tendency for it to decrease.

In spite of these compensatory changes the total peripheral resistance still falls on exposure to heat (Fig. 5–16). Thauer (1965) has suggested, on the basis of his own observations, that the view that changes in the resistance of blood vessels at the surface are compensated by vasoconstriction elsewhere needs revision. According to Thauer, peripheral resistance may be halved when ambient temperature rises from thermal neutrality to 40°C. If blood pressure is to be maintained, the cardiac output must then be increased.

Cardiac Output, Stroke Volume, and Pulse Rate

As expected from the argument above, cardiac output increases on exposure to temperature above the thermoneutral zone both in resting man (Scott et al., 1940) and in animals (Whittow, 1965, in the ox; Whittow

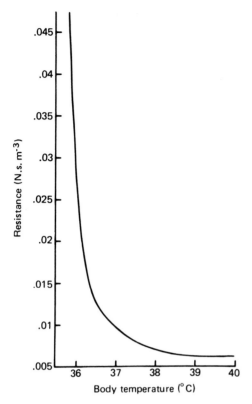

Fig. 5–16. Relation between total peripheral resistance and body temperature (Wezler and Thauer, 1943).

et al., 1964, for the chicken). In man, the output of the heart may reach as much as 15 liters/minute, more than would be expected from the increase in peripheral blood flow (Hertzmann, 1959). If the estimates for either cardiac output or total peripheral blood flow are not in serious error then there appears to be an increased blood flow to other parts of the body during heat exposure. Such an increased blood flow may well be associated, at least in part, with the increase in metabolism that occurs when body temperature is elevated.

The increase in cardiac output is made up by increases in both stroke volume and pulse rate, the contribution made by each varying according to species and the circumstances of the heat exposure. On exposure to a warm dry climate, the increase in car-

diac output in cattle is caused mainly by the increase in stroke volume. Under more severe heat stress, however, further increases in the output of the heart are associated with an increase in pulse rate, as in man. Moreover, in cattle, at least, the cardiovascular response to hyperthermia can be reproduced by local heating of the hypothalamus (Whittow, 1968).

If heat exposure is prolonged and body temperature rises to near the lethal limit, cardiac output falls again because of a decrease in stroke volume, whereas pulse rate remains high. At this point, it appears that there is not sufficient time for the heart to fill between each stroke, and the collapse of the circulatory system is imminent.

Blood Pressure

The diastolic blood pressure and mean blood pressure decrease in a warm ambient, whereas pulse rate increases in man and other animals. These changes occur in association with a decreased peripheral resistance and an increased cardiac output. Under more severe stress, when body core temperature is elevated, the systolic pressure tends to increase.

Blood Volume

It should be obvious from the above account that an increase in blood volume is of advantage on heat exposure and there is evidence to show that an increase does indeed occur. Experimental results, however, are somewhat conflicting because the extent to which blood volume can increase depends on the availability of water. The increase also tends to be greater when the subject exercises. Unacclimatized men may increase their blood volume by 10 percent (Robinson, 1963) when subjected to heat stress. On prolonged exposure the increase may be even greater. Dehydration during heat exposure must therefore be expected to have adverse effects related to the efficiency of the circulatory system as well as to limiting evaporative heat loss.

CHAPTER 6

Endocrine and Reproductive Systems

Because the endocrine system is concerned with the maintenance of the animal's internal environment in spite of changes in the external environment, it is to be expected that the system is influenced by changes in climatic conditions. The hormones associated with the control of metabolism, that is, those from the thyroid, adrenal cortex, and adrenal medulla, are especially likely to respond to changes in ambient temperature because of the changes that occur in metabolic rate, and the hormonal systems associated with the control of water and electrolyte balance are challenged during periods of high evaporative loss. The extent to which the other endocrine organs may be involved is not immediately evident, except that because the components of the endocrine system are closely interdependent, it is unlikely that one system can be changed without any influence on the rest. The literature on endocrinological aspects of exposure to high temperature has recently been comprehensively reviewed by Gale (1973) and by Collins and Weiner (1968), and previously by Berde (1951).

The Thyroid Gland

The secretion of thyroxine by the thyroid gland is controlled by the output of trophic hormone from the anterior hypophysis. This, in turn, depends partly on a feedback system directly to the pituitary by the circulating thyroxine and partly on the release of thyrotrophic releasing factor from the hypothalamus. There are therefore two possible ways in which the output of the gland can be influenced: either by variations in the level of circulating hormone or by some nervous mechanism. It is possible that both channels are involved in adjustments to changes in ambient temperature.

The techniques used to study the thyroid gland have evolved over many years. Older techniques have depended on examining sections of the thyroid gland and estimating the height of the epithelial cells. It is now possible to measure the rate at which radioactive iodine is taken up and released from the gland, the concentration of protein-bound iodine in blood, and the rate at which injected radioactive thyroxine disappears, as well as the actual concentration of thyroxine in plasma by means of a competitive binding assay. Unfortunately, many of the relevant studies were made before the development of the new methods, and even recent investigations have not employed the full range of measurements. Results must therefore be interpreted with care because a rise in the concentration of hormone in the blood may be the result of an increased rate of secretion, a decreased rate of utilization, or a change in blood volume. Studies on the release of thyroid stimulating hormone (TSH) have been restricted because a readily applied and reliable assay has not been available.

The bulk of investigations into the role of ambient temperature in regulating thyroid gland activity has been directed toward a study of the effects of low temperatures. Below the critical temperature, the secretion of thyroxine increases and comparisons made between high and low ambient temperatures have demonstrated differences in many species. Some studies have embraced the whole range of ambient temperatures, both below and above the critical temperature, and have demonstrated that not only is the activity of the thyroid gland increased in cold exposure by comparison with the thermally neutral temperatures, but it is also decreased in the warm. For example, in the rat, Dempsey and Astwood (1943) have estimated that the amount of thyroxine secreted is 9.5 μg at 1°C, 5.2 μg at 25°C, and only 1.7 μg at 35°C. Similar results have been reported for a number of species using different techniques. In the ox, Johnson and Ragsdale (1960) have found that the fall in thyroid activity is very abrupt at high temperatures (Fig. 6–1). The decline in the heat has also been shown in rams (Brook et al., 1962), pigeons and rabbits (Chaudhuri and Sadhu, 1961), mice (Hellmann and Collins, 1957), guinea pigs (Schmidt and Schmidt, 1938), poultry (Hoffman and Shaffner, 1950), and pigs (Ingram and Slebodzinski, 1965).

In a study over the whole lifespan of

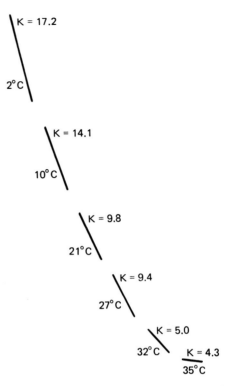

Fig. 6–1. The rate of release of radio iodine (measured as the K value) in cattle kept at various environmental temperatures. A large K value, indicating a rapid release of iodine, indicates a rapid release of hormone (redrawn from Johnson and Ragsdale, 1960).

the rat the position proved to be different (Johnson et al., 1966). Some rats were raised at 28°C and fed *ad libitum*; others were raised at 34°C and fed *ad libitum*. Still another group was kept at 28°C but was restricted in food intake to that which the 34°C group took. At first, the group at 34°C had a lower thyroid activity than the controls, but after 2 months the position was reversed, even though the rats at 34°C did not have a higher oxygen consumption. It was suggested that in this case the rate of degradation of thyroxine increased at high ambient temperatures and, therefore, that a rate of hormone secretion higher than in the control group was necessary.

In man there is also some evidence that thyroid activity is lower in the heat (Hare and Haigh, 1955; Goldberg et al.,

1964), although the view has been challenged. It appears, however (MacGregor and Loh, 1941), that after full corrections and allowances have been made there is a reduction in metabolism of about 5 percent in a tropical climate, although there is considerable individual variation and some people appear to exhibit no reduction at all. It is this extreme variability among individuals, combined with the differences in technique used, that probably accounts for some investigators having failed to find any difference in man after exposure to heat.

On exposure to cold, the increase in the amount of thyroxine secreted by the thyroid gland is believed to stimulate metabolism, and the depression of metabolism at high ambient temperatures appears to represent a type of chemical thermoregulation in the heat. It should be remembered that even a slight rise in body temperature is expected to increase metabolism because of the Arrhenius-Van't Hoff effect. Such an effect can be observed when man or animals are abruptly exposed to a hot environment. The decrease in thyroxine secretion, however, appears to offset this effect when enough time has been allowed at the higher ambient temperature for a new equilibrium of circulating hormone to be developed (Robinson, 1949).

Removal of the thyroid gland or treatment with such antithyroid substances as thiouracil tends to lower the body temperature and metabolic rate, with a resultant increase in heat tolerance. This experimental reduction in thyroid activity is analogous to the process that occurs naturally on exposure to heat. Ingram and Slebodzinski (1965) have found that thyroidectomized pigs that have been given a standard replacement dose of thyroxine fail to respond to 14 days at a high temperature by reducing metabolism as the controls do. Moreover, when such pigs are exposed to a thermoneutral temperature there are some signs of thyroid deficiency that are not seen at higher temperatures.

These studies suggest a controlling influence of thyroxine over the metabolic response to heat. Some investigators hold the view that the Arrhenius-Van't Hoff effect is also partly dependent on thyroxine when animals are suddenly subjected to a very hot environment. Donhoffer et al. (1953a,b) have suggested that in rats the rise in metabolism can largely be eliminated in animals that have been thyroidectomized, hypophysectomized, or treated with thiouracil. Some small effect of the thyroid may also be present in the increased metabolism of fever (Atkins, 1960), although the effect is not marked.

There have been claims by Mansfeld (1946) and Berde (1948) that the thyroid gland secretes a specific "cooling hormone" called "thermothyrin A." These workers believe that removal of the thyroid gland in fact decreases heat tolerance, but their claims do not appear to have been confirmed. Until more evidence is available, the existence of such a hormone must be held in considerable doubt.

A possible consequence of a reduced secretion of thyroxine under hot conditions, which is discussed by Collins and Weiner (1968), is that because growth largely depends on the permissive action of thyroxine, animals can be expected to grow slowly in a hot environment. Under experimental conditions there is a little evidence in some species to support this idea. However, whether animals in the tropics generally grow more slowly than in temperate climates has not been established.

The mechanisms by which the output of the thyroid gland is diminished in the heat are not yet fully understood. Explanations based on the feedback from the circulating level of thyroxine cannot be readily made. If the rate of thyroxine utilization is decreased in a warm environment, then a rise in the levels of thyroxine in the blood would be expected and the release of TSH by the pituitary would be suppressed by negative feedback. The expected result would be a decline in the production of thyroxine. However, if this is a true picture, some other mechanism that decreases the rate at which thyroxine is utilized must be involved. Another possibility is that some mechanism in the hypothalamus reduces signals to the pituitary; that is, less thyrotrophic hormone releasing factor is allowed to reach the pituitary and hence the production of TSH is reduced. Some evidence to support this view is provided by the work of Andersson (1964), who has shown that if the preoptic region of the hypothalamus is warmed in goats exposed to the cold, then the expected rise in thyroid hormone production is inhibited. What has yet to be established, however, is that there is normally a rise in brain temperature when the thyroid gland is suppressed on exposure to heat. In some instances this may be true, but there is evidence from studies on the pig (Ingram and Legge, 1971b) that on exposure to mild heat, body temperature actually falls before rising slightly.

In most species, body temperature tends to be a little higher in a hot environment than in a thermally neutral one, but a similar rise in temperature may also occur on exposure to moderate cold. It has also been demonstrated that cooling the hypothalamus leads to a diuresis and it is therefore possible that changes in hormone concentration which follow a change in temperature may be related, at least in part, to a change in blood volume (Evans and Ingram, 1974). Because experiments involving local heating or cooling of the brain are usually of a short duration, however, the interpretation of changes in hormone concentration in the blood must be made with great care.

The Adrenal Gland

Medullary Hormones

The hormones of the adrenal medulla include noradrenaline, which is also produced at certain nerve endings and acts as a transmitter substance. For the purpose of the present discussion, however, attention is restricted to the release of hormone into the blood stream from the adrenal gland.

On theoretical grounds, an appropriate response of the adrenal medulla when an animal is exposed to heat appears to be a decrease in the secretion of hormone, rather as in the case with the thyroid. At present, evidence on this point is lacking for most species, but in the horse there is strong evidence that secretion actually increases. In this species, the sweat glands respond to circulating adrenaline, which is in some respects rather surprising because this hormone also may be expected to raise the metabolism and cause a cutaneous vasoconstriction. Possibly, the quantities of hormone released at the onset of sweating are too small to have calorigenic effects, but investigations have not been made on this point.

In other species, also, the sweat glands respond to injections of adrenaline and noradrenaline. Under natural conditions, however, it is probable that the hormone is produced at the nerve ending very close to the sweat gland and destroyed before entering the general circulation.

Glucocorticoids

Adrenalectomized rats succumb to high environmental temperatures more easily than do controls and are to some extent protected by extracts of the adrenal gland (Hermanson and Hartman, 1945). It therefore appears that the gland is of importance at both ends of the temperature extreme, for the sensitivity of adrenalectomized animals to cold stress is well established. Further evidence of the glands' involvement in the response to acute exposure to high temperature derives from studies on its ascorbic acid content, which is much reduced in rats 1 hour after exposure to 38°C (Sayers and Sayers, 1947). Increases are found in the plasma 17-

hydroxycorticosteroids of the anesthetized dog the body temperature of which is raised by external heating (Richards and Egdahl, 1956). Because the same result is not obtained in hypophysectomized animals, the response must involve the pituitary. This idea is further strengthened by the studies of Chowers et al. (1966), who have found that cortisol levels increase in the conscious dog when the preoptic region is heated locally.

Prolonged exposure to high temperatures under natural conditions, however, appears to be associated with a decrease in glucocorticoid activity in a number of species, including man (Collins and Weiner, 1968). In terms of a reduced rate of metabolism in a warm climate, this response is easier to understand than an increase. Some of the increase in adrenal cortical activity that occurs after sudden exposure to a hot environment may in fact be a response to a stress rather than a specific response to the heat. The transient effects of injections of adrenocortical hormones to animals subjected to a hot environment, moreover, may be part of the general protection to stress given by these hormones. The possibility that the glucocorticoids contribute to the animals' ability to withstand heat via their secondary role of affecting electrolytes should not be overlooked, however.

Mineralocorticoids

The problems involved in the production of large quantities of sweat have been indicated (Chapter 4) in relation to salt and water balance, particularly in man, who can produce 12 liters/day. Similar problems, however, occur to a lesser extent in other animals exposed to hot climates and forced to evaporate moisture. In cattle, for example, some fluid and electrolytes may be lost through drooling, which occurs during severe heat stress, in addition to the water loss

through panting. It is therefore to be expected that the adrenocortical hormones concerned in electrolyte balance are involved in the response to exposure to hot climates.

The principal mineralocorticoid is aldosterone, which accounts for about two-thirds of the total sodium-retaining activity of the adrenal hormones, whereas the other one-third is exercised by the glucocorticoids. The actions of the glucocorticoids on the kidney are complex, however, because they tend to increase glomerular filtration rate and initial sodium loss, on the one hand, and to promote the later reabsorption of sodium, on the other. In addition, the glucocorticoids influence the distribution of electrolytes and water between extra- and intracellular pools and probably play a role in the expansion of the extracellular fluid volume that occurs during acclimatization to heat.

It has been shown that exposure to a hot environment leads to an increase in aldosterone in the urine of man (Collins et al., 1955), but the extent to which the increase occurs is related not so much to heat exposure itself as to the amount of sweating that takes place. As pointed out (Chapter 4), human sweat contains a high proportion of salt. As it is known that aldosterone output increases during salt deficiency and decreases on salt loading, it is probable that the rise in aldosterone excretion in the heat is related to the loss of sodium. In fact, if salt and water deficiency is prevented during work and sweating at high temperatures, no increase in aldosterone occurs.

Even though the evidence suggests that the loss of sodium stimulates the release of aldosterone, O'Connor (1962) has drawn attention to other mechanisms that control salt loss and that may be even more important on initial exposure to heat. For example, the loss of sodium in sweat leads to a decrease in extracellular fluid, which in turn brings about an increase in the concentration of plasma protein. The result of this is a decreased glomerular filtration rate and a reduction in sodium loss, all of which occurs without the intervention of hormonal control. As Collins and Weiner (1968) have suggested, the role of aldosterone may be in the long-term adjustments of salt and water balance on exposure to heat.

As already mentioned, if men are kept in salt and water balance, there is no change in aldosterone output even after several days exposure to heat. Macfarlane (1963) has discussed the possibility that an increase in environmental temperature may itself influence aldosterone output, but there is no conclusive evidence in support of this idea. Nevertheless, it is possible to demonstrate an increase in the amount of aldosterone in the urine during the summer over that in winter months (Yoshimura, 1960), even though salt balance has been established. The mechanisms involved are not clear, however, because acclimatization to heat involves an increase in blood volume and in extracellular fluid, whereas the stimulus for increase in aldosterone secretion is a fall in blood volume. One possibility, suggested by Yoshimura (1960), is that the central blood volume decreases while an expansion occurs in the peripheral parts of the vascular system.

Under the influence of aldosterone, the sodium concentration of sweat is reduced, but this fall in sodium loss takes some 6 hours to develop. Part of the time lag is accounted for by the mechanism of aldosterone action, which involves protein synthesis in the nucleus as has been demonstrated in the toad bladder. The time taken for this synthesis is 1–3 hours and fully explains the delay observed with respect to the kidney tubules. The additional time taken for an effect to be manifest on the sweat glands may be related to the rather low oxygen concentration. Sweat glands are known to contain large amounts of lactic acid, which suggests an anerobic metabolic pathway for glycogen, whereas aldosterone requires aerobic conditions (Collins and Weiner, 1968). Aldosterone may also reduce the quantity of sweat produced by the glands. If men are

allowed to acclimatize to heat while in salt deficiency, the extra capacity to sweat they acquire may be offset by a rise in aldosterone secretion.

In other animals, the salt loss from sweating is not as severe as in man. The donkey may lose nearly 8 percent of its body weight during a day in the desert but there is no corresponding loss of sodium; a similar state is true of the camel. Macfarlane (1963, 1964) has studied sheep exposed to high temperatures and has found that, as in man, urine flow is reduced after a few hours. However, there is an increase in sodium loss, and the more severe the dehydration, the higher the Na/K ratio in the urine. Meanwhile, the excretion of aldosterone remains unchanged. It is only during rehydration, when the extracellular fluid expands, that the secretion of aldosterone is stimulated and sodium is retained. In panting animals, exposure to heat leads to a loss of water and sodium is left behind; however, under very severe conditions, quantities of saliva containing sodium may be drooled from the mouth. When a similar situation is created experimentally by exteriorizing the duct of the parotid salivary gland in goats, the loss of sodium leads to aldosterone secretion and a lowering of the Na/K ratio in the saliva, although the threshold for sodium retention by the salivary glands is much higher than that for the kidney. Under very severe heat load, therefore, drooling may be a further complicating factor in the stimulation of aldosterone secretion.

Antidiuretic Hormone

Exposure to a hot environment in man and animals leads to an increase in water retention that may in some instances be even greater than the additional evaporative loss. The result is that after an initial water deficit both the extracellular volume and the blood volume increase (Robinson, 1949; Yoshimura, 1960). At first, the reduction in urine flow on exposure to heat may be related entirely to a reduced glomerular filtration rate (GFR) consequent on a lower renal blood flow and dehydration in both man and animals (Macfarlane, 1964; Radigan and Robinson, 1949). However, after a period of time the GFR increases again (Pitesky and Last, 1951).

The longer-term reduction in urine flow during heat exposure is related to an increase in the levels of antidiuretic hormone (ADH), even when there is a positive water balance (Collins and Weiner, 1968). In man (Hellmann and Weiner, 1953) working in a hot environment, ADH in the plasma increases. There is a similar increase in sheep (Macfarlane, 1963, 1964) subjected to water deprivation in summer. Moreover, in both man and sheep, a standard heat exposure in summer is followed by a greater rise in ADH secretion than in winter (Macfarlane and Robinson, 1957) probably because there is a seasonal difference in the availability of water in the body spaces, which in turn depends on salt balance. The injection of vasopressin into the sheep and camel, however, leads to an unexpected increase in urine flow and in the secretion of sodium and potassium. According to Schmidt-Nielsen (1964), this is possibly because the vasopressin is given when urine flow is already low and therefore causes an increase in the excretion of electrolytes, which carry water with them. However, others believe this indicates that ADH is not responsible for the lower urine production in these animals.

When dehydrated and exposed to heat the camel reduces its amount of sweat loss, and the possibility has been raised that this also occurs in man. The evidence for reduced sweat production except in very severe dehydration in man is poor, however; nor is there any evidence that the injection of pituitrin or vasopressin reduces sweat secretion.

It has been demonstrated that the secretion of ADH can be controlled by osmoreceptors in the hypothalamus, which raises the question of whether it can also be influenced by temperature in the hypothalamus. Itoh (1954) believes from experiments on the rat that there is enough evidence to support the idea, but others disagree. There is some evidence, however, that local cooling of the hypothalamus can decrease the quantity of ADH released and that local heating can produce an increase. It has also been suggested that blood volume changes may influence secretion, and there is evidence for the existence of volume receptors connected with ADH release. It is likely that modification in ADH release on exposure to hot climates depends on changes in osmotic pressure, but it is evident from the discussion above that some other mechanism may also be involved.

Reproduction

Male

The best-known effect of temperature on reproduction concerns the sensitivity of the mammalian testis, and the subject has recently been reviewed by Waites (1970). If these organs are confined experimentally or by natural accident to the abdomen, or if they are insulated with a nonconductive material, then degenerative changes occur. The most developed germ cells are first affected and the process gradually involves all stages down to spermatogonia. The germinal epithelium is finally affected, although the Leydig cells are less affected and are believed to continue, at least for a while, to secrete androgens. In most mammals, the testes are housed in the scrotum, which, being outside the abdomen and also being supplied with sweat glands, is at a temperature about 5°C lower than the rectal temperature (Waites and Moule, 1961). In some animals, however, for example, elephants and whales, the testes are housed in the abdomen. In addition, the blood supply to the testes passes through the pampiniform plexus, in which arteries and veins are applied closely together along a tortuous path that allows the cool blood returning from the scrotum to reduce the temperature of the arterial supply. Damage to this structure, for example by cadmium, leads to testicular damage similar to that caused by heating. According to Waites and Setchell (1964), a rise in testicular temperature leads to an increase in oxygen consumption by the tissues but not to an increase in blood flow; consequently, hypoxia develops.

An additional mechanism that helps to maintain a testicular temperature below that deep in the body is the reaction of the tunica dartos muscle of the scrotum (Phillips and McKenzie, 1934). On exposure to heat, the muscle relaxes and allows the testes to become fully dependent. This not only allows a 20 percent greater surface area for heat exchange but also extends the pampiniform plexus and so probably improves the heat exchange process there.

Experiments on rams and on small laboratory mammals have shown that even exposures to high temperatures of less than an hour may cause damage to sperm. In rams exposed to 40°C for between 6 hours and 3 days, the decrease in semen quality is proportional to the length of exposure. The decrease first appears in semen ejaculated 13–21 days later and lasts 35–39 days (Moule and Waites, 1963). It is therefore apparent that even short exposures to high temperatures during the hottest part of the day may be sufficient to reduce fertility. In man, it is possible that a hot bath, or even the wearing of closefitting underclothes during warm weather, may damage stored sperm.

Female

The effects of a hot climate on reproduction in female mammals have been studied by Macfarlane et al. (1959). Exposure of pregnant females to high temperature leads to an increase in the incidence of fetal resorption that is only partly accounted for by the lower intake of protein and vitamins in the heat. Injections of thyroxine help to reduce the number of fetuses lost but the loss is still greater than in controls. Acclimatization before mating has no significant effect on fetal mortality, but the incidence of ovulation is reduced, at least in rats.

Macfarlane and his colleagues have studied a colony of rats raised for several generations at a high temperature. They have taken care to adjust for any possible vitamin deficiency that may occur as a result of a lower food intake in a hot environment. They have found that even when the females are mated with males raised in a cool environment the number that become pregnant is smaller than in a control group. This may be partly because of a failure to implant, for they have also shown that failure to implant is more common in a hot environment. Resorption of fetuses persists even after several generations in the heat.

Fertility of Groups

The factors influencing the fertility of groups of animals removed from their natural habitats are very complex. It appears from the above evidence, however, that at least part of the observed fall in human fertility in hot climates may be related to the direct effect of temperature on the reproductive system. In both Australia and the southern United States, the conception rate among white people who originate in a more temperate climate is lower during the sum-

mer months. Animals and human popula-
tions indigenous to the tropics obviously
manage to survive and even increase in
number. Little is known about whether their
reproductive ability can be enhanced in a
cooler climate, however, because direct
transfer almost always involves other limiting factors.

CHAPTER 7

Behavior

Although many animals have special mechanisms that enable them to control their body temperatures, such as sweating, panting, and shivering, these activities involve the use of materials that may be in short supply, such as water in a desert climate. Modifications of behavior patterns, however, may be sufficient to enable an animal to survive a potential environmental stress without involving these other mechanisms. The most obvious and well-developed patterns of behavioral thermoregulation are perhaps exhibited by man, who in all but the most primitive tribes varies the amount of clothing he wears and, in the more highly developed societies, employs air conditioning systems that make him almost totally independent of the climate.

Behavioral patterns related to climatic conditions may also be observed among less highly developed animals, however, and in these instances they are likely to be the sole means by which the animal manages to survive. For example, Edney (1957) has demonstrated that although the woodlouse has no control over its water loss and is limited to living in humid conditions, it can nevertheless survive in the hot desert. Closer investigation has shown that the animal inhabits burrows under the sand, where the climatic conditions are similar to those encountered by woodlice in England. In this instance, the simple selection of a microclimate has enabled an animal to survive in what at first appear to be lethal conditions (Fig. 7–1). A similar selection of a microclimate also occurs in amphibia that live in the desert and that can become dehydrated very rapidly away from shelter (Warburg, 1972).

Avoidance of Adverse Conditions

The avoidance of adverse conditions is to some extent exhibited by most animals and can be observed even in simple organisms. If ciliates or planaria, for example, are placed in a long tube, one end of which

91

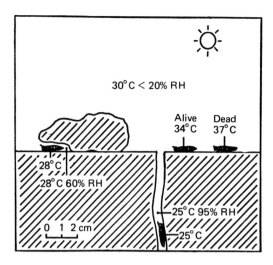

Fig. 7–1. Body temperature of woodlice in various positions in the desert. The animal in the burrow is in a relatively cool environment that is nearly saturated with water (Edney, 1957).

is heated and the other cooled, the creatures avoid the extremes of temperature and congregate at some point in the middle. When the distances between an animal's habitat and the adverse conditions are great, behavior of this sort simply leads to the exclusion of a species from certain geographical regions. The selection of favorable climatic conditions may also operate over small distances, however, as in the case of the woodlouse, and is particularly employed by small insects and annelids (Cloudsley-Thompson and Chadwick, 1964). Seasonal migration of animals may also involve a degree of thermoregulatory behavior, although such other factors as the availability of food usually complicate the issue.

An additional way in which an animal may avoid adverse conditions without moving to another region is by becoming dormant. In winter, such periods of dormancy are termed "hibernation," and the corresponding term during the summer is "estivation." Animals that estivate usually select some part of the territory that is protected from the heat, such as a burrow, where temperature fluctuations are much reduced. Activity is reduced to the minimum with a correspondingly small heat load to be dissipated.

Again, this type of behavior is usually associated not only with the avoidance of heat but also with a shortage of food. For example, the Californian pocket mouse (Tucker, 1962) and the kangaroo rat undergo periods of torpor during the day at any time of the year when food is in short supply, and the period of torpor is increased if the food supply is further reduced. In these animals, estivation appears to be associated with surviving food shortages, which in turn are usually a direct consequence of climatic conditions, particularly water shortage. Estivation is then perhaps to be regarded more as an adaptation to the adverse conditions of a hot dry climate in general than as a specific mechanism of thermoregulation.

Long periods of dormancy may also occur in invertebrates subjected to hot dry conditions. In these species, too, estivation appears to serve a function similar to that seen in higher animals. Snails have been studied in the hot desert by Cloudsley-Thompson and Chadwick (1964) and by Schmidt-Nielsen et al. (1971). These animals manage to survive periods of several months or even years of exposure on the desert floor simply by sealing themselves into the shell and reducing metabolism and water loss to the minimum. It has been calculated that, aided by the white color of the shell, which reflects much of the radiant heat, a snail can survive for 4 years in this condition (Fig. 7–2). Once the rain falls and plants begin to grow again, the animals become active and replenish their food and water supplies. Earthworms may also estivate in burrows during the summer months, although for these creatures it is the humidity rather than the temperature itself that is the more important factor.

The life cycles of insects may include a period of dormancy called "diapause," during which the animal is particularly resistant to heat and desiccation as well as to cold. It is therefore not surprising to find

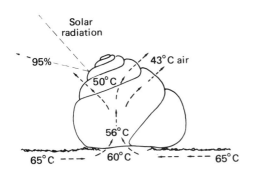

Fig. 7–2. Distribution of temperatures around a snail on the desert floor. Arrows indicate direction of heat flow (Schmidt-Nielsen et al., 1971).

that insects inhabiting the hot dry parts of the world have a diapause during the driest season. Many other invertebrates and protozoa produce eggs that are resistant to adverse conditions. They may also be able to encase themselves in cysts. Moreover, the production of such resistant forms may be induced by the onset of adverse climatic conditions. In some instances, such adaptations as the production of resistant eggs only ensure the survival of the species and the adult individual perishes.

So far, attention has been focused on animals that either avoid living in adverse conditions or that "shut off" their activity for relatively long periods, measured at the shortest in terms of days. Most creatures, however, have periods of activity that occur in regular cycles associated with day and night. One very simple method for an animal to avoid the heat of the day is to be nocturnal and spend the day in a burrow, which remains much cooler than the desert surface. The jerboa (Kirmiz, 1962) is one example of a small desert mammal that spends the day in a burrow. Some lizards and snakes are also nocturnal, although certain deserts have very cold nights, which may provide climatic conditions just as unsuitable at the opposite extreme for so called "cold-blooded" animals.

Creatures that remain nocturnal whether

the daylight hours are hot or temperate are, of course, genetically fixed in their habit, but some species actually change their activity according to the climatic conditions. Cattle, particularly those from temperate zones, normally graze during the daytime but when they are transported to the tropics their behavior is modified. According to Seath and Millar (1946), the extent to which the change in behavior occurs depends on air temperature, solar radiation, and body temperature. For example, cattle spend 11 percent of the time grazing during the daytime when the dry bulb temperature is 29°C, but during the night, when air temperature is still 27°C and solar radiation obviously nil, the cattle graze for 35 percent of the time.

Among diurnal animals, one obvious response to intense heat is to seek a shaded area, with its reduced load from solar radiation. Behavior of this sort is evident in many species, including man, and can again be seen among European cattle in the tropics, or even in temperate regions on a hot day. A simple selection of any shaded area, however, is not necessarily the best solution to the problem facing the animal. As Schmidt-Nielsen (1964) has pointed out, the jackrabbit (Fig. 7–3) greatly increases its capacity to lose heat by selecting a shaded position in which the large radiator-like ears can be exposed to blue sky, where the radiant temperature is considerably lower than

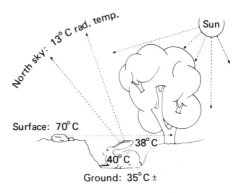

Fig. 7–3. Distribution of temperatures and directions of heat flow around a jackrabbit lying in the shade (Schmidt-Nielsen, 1964).

that of the surrounding ground and solid objects. By contrast, although the shade provided by a metal roof may reduce solar radiation, if the roof is at a higher temperature than the skin, the animal still gains heat. Shade-seeking behavior can also be observed in reptiles and birds, which tend to retreat out of the sun during the hottest part of the day. When disturbed, snakes may sometimes attempt to follow the shade provided by a man's shadow as he moves about, an action that is easily misinterpreted!

In the absence of shade provided by the environment itself, birds may protect their young from intense heat by holding out their wings, or they may protect their eggs by shading them with their bodies. Under cloudy skies, masked boobies incubating their eggs orient themselves at random with respect to the position of the sun; under a clear sky, however, they move round with the sun, keeping the shade provided by their bodies over the eggs (Bartholomew, 1964). Birds also have an additional dimension in which to escape the heat. Under hot conditions the larger species have been observed to fly up to a height of 700–1000 m, where they remain all day soaring on the air currents. At this height, the air temperature is much cooler than near the ground.

The Effect of Postural Changes

Changes in posture or in orientation to the sun's rays and the periodic selection of a shaded position may be employed by some animals in such a way as to relieve the strain placed on special thermoregulatory mechanisms. In other instances, behavior may be the sole means by which body temperature can be regulated.

As mentioned, the jackrabbit makes maximum use of its ears as radiators by

selecting a shaded area that is open to the sky. A similar device of exposing a well-vascularized surface to a relatively low radiant temperature is also employed by some birds. Bartholomew (1964), in a discussion of homeostasis in the desert environment, has described how young Laysan albatross orient themselves with their backs to the sun and then stand on their heels, so that the highly vascularized surfaces of the web feet can be spread out just above the ground in the shade provided by the body. The amount of solar radiation falling on the body may also be controlled, even in the absence of shade, by changing the angle the body makes with the sun rays. Among insects, the locust has been found to employ this device, which may make as much as 6°C difference to the body temperature (Stower and Griffiths, 1966). Lizards also pay particular attention to the orientation of their bodies to the sun (Templeton, 1970). The effect of changes in position can be examined by taking a model animal (Fig. 7–4) and observing the shadow it casts when illuminated by a focused light beam representing the sun. The greater the area of shadow, the greater the surface that is directly illuminated (of course, the system does not work when the sun is directly overhead). Moreover, the animal's choice of an indirect surface to stand on may also modify the angle at which the sun's rays strike the body and so determine the amount of radiant energy received (White, 1973). The effective radiative surface of the body may also be modified by spreading the limbs or by holding them close to the body, as has been demonstrated in the pig (Mount, 1968a).

Adjustments of convective heat loss may be achieved simply by moving the body. For example, the young albatross described above rock on their heels and so flap their feet in the air. A similar effect is achieved by the African elephant when it gently moves its large, well-vascularized ears and so increases the air movement over their surface. During flight, birds may make use of the

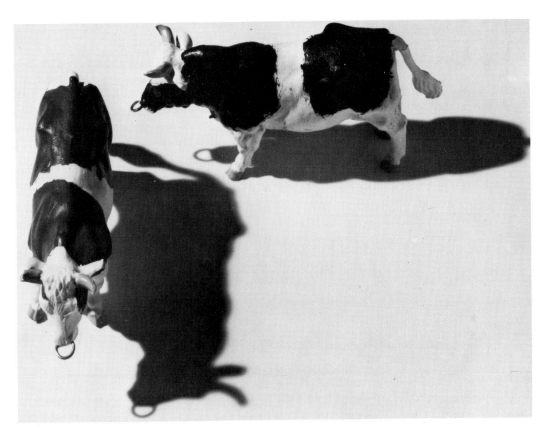

Fig. 7–4. Effect of changes in orientation to the sun on the radiant heat load. The model animals have been illuminated by a lamp set at an angle of 30° to represent the sun. The area of the shadow cast indicates the area of the body receiving radiation.

convective cooling provided as they move through the air, as for example when the budgerigar extends the unfeathered parts of its feet and limbs in the slipstream, an action that only occurs at air temperatures over 36°C.

Seals are another set of animals that sometimes enhance the degree of convective cooling. These creatures often live in very cold water and are protected from excessive heat loss by the thick layer of subcutaneous fat. Once out of the water during warm weather, however, the insulation that protected them against the cold now tends to make them hyperthermic. In these circumstances, the seal may be seen to raise its body partly off the ground and to wave its well-vascularized flippers in the air, or to lie on land with its tail flipper in the water.

Conductive heat transfer, either with the ground or with other animals, may also control an appreciable part of the heat balance. Such animals as pigs, kittens, chickens, and some lizards, which huddle together in the cold and so reduce heat loss, separate and lie apart when the temperature rises above the critical value (Fig. 7–5). Observations on the pig have also demonstrated that the animal's posture changes with ambient temperature, allowing minimal contact with the floor under cold conditions but maximum contact when the air temperature is high. Cooling the body by contact with the ground is employed by such animals as the antelope ground squirrel, which presses its body against the ground in its relatively cool bur-

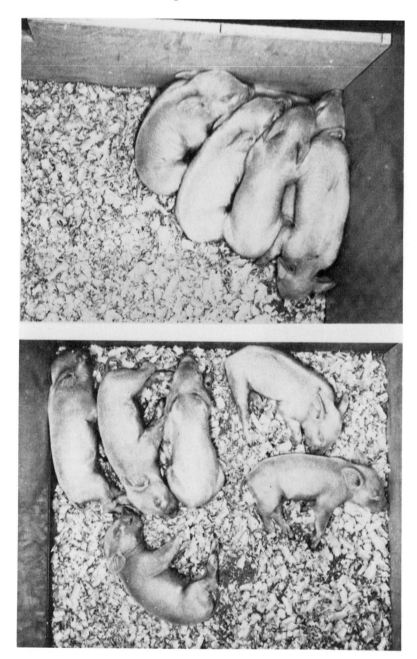

Fig. 7–5. Group of pigs in cool (top) and warm (bottom) conditions (from Mount, 1968a).

row, or by lizards, which pause during a journey across the desert floor to wriggle themselves into the cooler layers of sand just below the surface and then press the abdomen down. Conversely, if the ground is hotter than the air the lizard may hold its body off the ground. The extent to which this happens is related to the temperature of the ground (De Witt, 1971) (Fig. 7–6).

Conductive and convective cooling may also be achieved by bathing in water, and, because the animal must subsequently dry off, bathing also involves evaporative cooling.

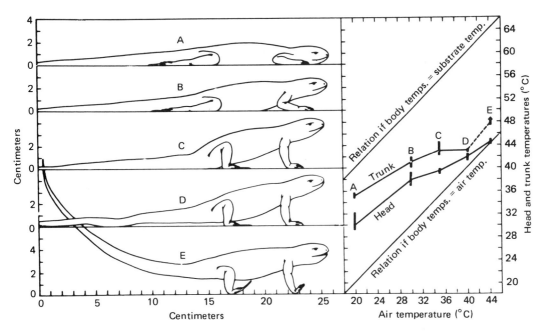

Fig. 7–6. Postures and steady-state temperatures of a lizard in relation to air and substrate temperatures (DeWitt, 1971; Courtesy of Masson et Cie, Paris).

Evaporative Heat Loss

When the temperature of the surroundings is close to body temperature, cooling can only be achieved to any extent by evaporation of water. This is achieved behaviorally in several ways by nonsweating animals. One adaptation involves wallowing in mud or water, and among the domestic animals the pig is well known for this type of behavior. Furthermore, because the pig has little hair, the water that evaporates from the surface probably derives most of the necessary latent heat from the body itself. Under conditions of extreme heat other animals may also wallow, but if the body is covered with a thick layer of hair the water or mud is likely to adhere to the ends of the hairs while the actual skin remains relatively dry. Under these conditions, a large part of the necessary latent heat may be derived from the ambient air, and the amount of cooling achieved is thus correspondingly reduced. This is of course not to say that

wallowing by a furred animal is of no practical use in cooling the body, only that its efficiency is reduced.

Where water is not available in any quantity, fluid for evaporation may be derived from the body itself. The rat wets its fur and feet with saliva under severe heat stress and the copious flow of saliva from cattle and pigs stressed by high temperatures may also increase evaporative loss provided it falls on the body. This method of cooling is of limited value, however, for in large animals much of the saliva falls on the ground and simply increases water loss without cooling. Moreover, small animals, such as the rat, have a very limited supply of water in the body. The survival value of fur licking for small rodents should not be dismissed, however. If the periods of severe heat are infrequent and of only short duration, this behavior pattern can allow a species to survive in a habitat in which it may otherwise perish.

Other sources of liquid in the body are the urine and feces, both of which are used as a wallow by several species. The wood-stalk, however, has developed a behavior pattern during heat stress of deliberately urinating down its naked legs and so evaporating the water directly from the skin surface, where most of the latent heat is derived from the body.

Evaporative loss cannot usually be employed by invertebrates because their small size limits the quantity of water available. Bees, however, use evaporative cooling in the control of hive temperature in the region occupied by the developing eggs. When the temperature can no longer be controlled by the combined action of the worker bees beating the wings and so providing an air stream through the hive, the workers bring in drops of water and spread them over the combs containing the developing egg cells.

Effectiveness of Behavioral Patterns in Regulating Body Temperature

It is now better appreciated that the reptiles and lower vertebrates are not "cold-blooded" animals, the body temperature of which follows that of the environment. Indeed, they are often found to have remarkably stable body temperatures, appreciably higher than the ambient air. In the absence of the highly developed thermoregulatory mechanisms seen in birds and mammals, behavior often accounts for most of this ability to maintain a steady temperature. According to studies by Bogert and Cowles (1959), some lizards are able to keep to their body temperature within a range of 2.5°C for 80 percent of the time by using the sort of behavior mentioned above (i.e., choice of position, orientation to the sun, and conductive cooling to the ground). Similar conclusions have been drawn by De Witt (1971).

Many mammals have either sweat glands or panting mechanisms that function in hot environments, but small mammals do not share this advantage. Nevertheless, such animals as the antelope ground squirrel survive in spite of being diurnal. This remarkable animal can tolerate a body temperature of 43°C and makes full use of this property by moving about over desert in the heat of the day and allowing its body temperature to approach lethal limits. Only at this point does it retire into its burrow and employ conductive cooling to the ground to reduce its temperature to about 38°C. As soon as this is achieved, it again runs out into the desert and begins the cycle all over again. The storage of heat is used by the camel and other large animals. They gain heat during the day and lose it again at night when it is cooler, so that no special behavior is involved. In the case of the antelope ground squirrel, however, the stored heat must be lost in the hot part of the day.

The behavior of the bee in controlling the temperature of the hive has already been mentioned and is of vital importance for the developing eggs and larvae. Under cold conditions, the worker bees cover the comb cells with their bodies, forming an insulative blanket. At higher temperatures, they employ fanning and the evaporation of water to cool the hive. The behavior, moreover, is sufficiently well organized to maintain the temperature of the developing larvae between 34°C and 35°C (Wigglesworth, 1965; Frisch, 1955).

Although clothing is often regarded as a separate subject, it is a form of behavioral thermoregulation. The choice of long flowing robes by inhabitants of the desert is important. Such clothing protects the skin from heat gain from solar radiation and still allows the evaporation of water in the form of sweat. Man, however, is particularly well equipped to regulate body temperature. Even in the total absence of clothing, the aborigines manage to survive in the Australian desert, which is hot by day and cold at night.

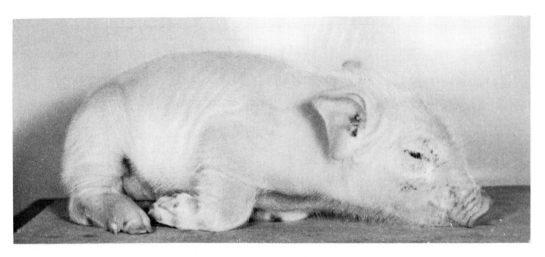

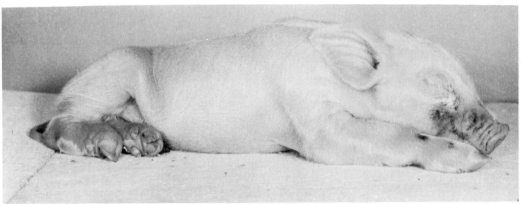

Fig. 7–7. Change in posture of a single pig in a cool (upper) and warm (lower) environment (Mount, 1968a).

Measurement of the Effects of Posture and Behavioral Patterns on Heat Loss

In the previous sections it has been shown that behavioral patterns can be effective in allowing animals to survive unpromising climatic conditions. In order to understand the role of behavior better, however, it is necessary to determine quantitatively the extent to which it modifies heat loss or gain. Pigs have received more attention than most animals in this respect. It has been shown (Mount, 1968a) that when young pigs change position from one in which the limbs

are held close to the body to one in which they are spread out, the effective area from which both radiation and convection can occur also changes (Fig. 7–7).

In these studies, the animal's oxygen consumption was measured while the animal was exposed in a chamber where the air temperature and the radiant temperature of the walls could be varied independently. The estimate derived from these studies is that the effective radiating surface of the pig increased from 67 to 76 percent of the total surface area as the air temperature increased from 20°C to 30°C and the animal spread out its limbs. At the same time as the change in posture occurred with increase in temperature, there was also an increase in blood flow in the skin. The surface temperature consequently rose, which also led to the increase of heat loss. Calculation showed that a third of the change in heat loss could be attributed to the effect of posture.

The effects of changes in position on convective heat loss are less easily determined. When the air in the chamber is kept as still as possible, natural convection currents caused by the heat of the animal's body are responsible for most of the air movement. Mount (1968a) has calculated that the effective convective area of the young pig changes from 76 to 86 percent of the total area as the animal stretches out its limbs when the temperature is raised from 20°C to 30°C. As is to be expected, the surface from which convection occurs is greater than that from which radiation takes place. This is simply because where two body surfaces face each other, for example, between the legs, radiative exchange can occur only between the skin surfaces but convective exchange can still occur with the air.

When there is forced convection from a stream of air in the chamber, measurements are much more difficult to make. Under these conditions the movement of air over the body is far from constant, as shown by Alexander (1961) in the lamb, and depends on the animal's orientation to the wind. In the pig, when air movement is measured from a localized area of the trunk, the rate of heat loss is proportional to the square root of the air velocity (Mount and Ingram, 1964). No such clearcut relation holds when heat loss from the whole animal is plotted against the average air movement in the chamber, however (Mount, 1968a). Under these conditions, heat loss is less than expected on the basis of the results obtained from a localized area. The discrepancy is probably related to the effects of posture and the markedly unequal distribution of air velocities over the animal's surface.

Heat loss by conduction becomes of importance when animals lie down, either to sleep or deliberately in an attempt to increase heat loss. Again, the problem has been investigated in the young pig, using a specially designed gradient layer mat that can be placed on any surface and at a number of different environmental temperatures. A change in posture, from one in which the animal lies on its own limbs with the body off the ground to one in which a large area of the trunk is in contact with the floor (see Fig. 7–7), is accompanied by an increase in thermal conductance to the floor of up to 50 percent. Under the conditions of the study, conduction still accounts for only 15 percent of the total, but under other conditions where the floor is colder than the air it could clearly account for a much greater proportion of the total.

The effect of wallowing in mud or water on the evaporation of water from the trunk has been studied under laboratory conditions by means of a ventilated sweat capsule. In the pig, evaporative moisture loss from the trunk, which has been wetted with clear water, increases from about 30 to 800 $gm.m^{-2}.h^{-1}$. After about 15 minutes, the rate begins to decline. If the body surface is smeared with mud, however, a similar rate of water loss is achieved and it persists for about 2 hours. A short visit to a mud wallow three or four times a day may therefore be all that is needed to maintain a rate of cutaneous vaporization similar to that of man, who sweats most efficiently.

The above examples have all been drawn from the pig, but similar demonstrations are possible for a variety of animals. In man, the effect of posture on heat loss has been clearly demonstrated by experiments involving the use of a rapidly responding gradient layer calorimeter (Benzinger et al., 1958). When a nude man adopts a flexed posture, there is an immediate fall in heat loss. When the body is relaxed the stored heat is released with the result that heat loss increases above the control level before declining again. Similar changes can be demonstrated when large animals change their position while in a gradient layer calorimeter.

Studies Involving a Choice of Environment by the Animal

One method of studying an animal's choice of environment under laboratory conditions is to use some sort of thermocline. At its simplest, this can take the form of a long tube heated at one end and cooled at the other. More complicated varieties employ a series of intercommunicating chambers in which the ambient conditions can be controlled.

Among the lower vertebrates the temperature selected appears to depend, at least to some extent, on the temperature to which the animal has previously been exposed. In studies of the carp, reviewed by Fry and Hochacka (1970), the fishes tend to select a water temperature close to that to which they have been acclimated. In studies carried out by different workers, using similar acclimation temperatures, however, the actual temperature selected has displayed an appreciable variation, suggesting that factors other than the thermal history also have an effect on the animal's choice of ambient conditions. One such factor is the season of the

year, or at least the changing length of day. Amphibia have also been tested in thermoclines and exhibit similar tendencies to select a temperature close to that to which they have been acclimated.

The temperature preferred by reptiles (see Templeton, 1970) may change over a 24-hour period. Diurnal lizards choose to rest in a cool temperature at night and a warmer one during the day. Temperature preference in reptiles is also complicated in some species by an apparently paradoxical effect of acclimation. For example, Willcroft and Anderson (1960) have found that lizards acclimated to a low environmental temperature select conditions that result in a higher body temperature than does another group acclimated to a high environmental temperature.

Mammals also display temperature preferences but, because of the highly developed mechanisms by which body temperature can be controlled, it is to be expected that they may more readily ignore the optimal conditions. In a study of young pigs, Mount (1963) has used a thermocline with four chambers giving a range of 23°–37°C, the critical temperature of the newborn pig being about 34°C. The animals tend to select the compartment at 30°C, but all the compartments are occupied by some individuals (Table 7–1). It has been concluded from this study that thermal comfort cannot nec-

Table 7–1. Ambient Temperatures Preferred by Young Pigs, both Singly and in Groups of Five; Numbers Choosing Different Temperatures[a]

Age of pigs (days)	Ambient temperature (°C)				Mean ± S.E. temperature (°C)
	23–28	29–31	32–34	35–37	
Single pigs					
<1	1	2	5	2	32.3 ± 0.94
1–7	8	16	4	0	29.3 ± 0.44
8–41	16	33	11	6	29.8 ± 0.64
Groups					
2–7	2	3	3	0	30.1 ± 1.03
8–41	3	9	4	1	30.4 ± 0.66

[a] From Mount (1963) by permission.

essarily be predicted within close limits by reference to the critical temperature as determined under laboratory conditions. A similar conclusion has been drawn from a study of pigs observed outdoors at all seasons of the year, in a natural environment consisting of woodland and pasture with access to shelter (Ingram and Legge, 1970b). In this study the animals show a strong tendency to avoid the most windy part of the enclosure, but they do not seek shelter in the hut until the ambient temperature is well below the critical value. At the higher end of the temperature scale, however, the sow, as a larger and more heat-susceptible animal, regularly seeks even a small area of shade.

obtained. The first studies of behavioral thermoregulation have involved placing the animal in a cold environment. As it moves about the cage, sooner or later, by accident, it makes the selected response (e.g., pressing a lever) and a reinforcement of a brief period of heating follows. After a period of time in this situation an animal begins to make regular responses and is said to be trained. Conversely, it has been possible to train animals in a hot environment to make a response that is followed by the reinforcement of some sort of cooling. The work on operant conditioning and behavioral thermoregulation has recently been reviewed by Corbit (1970).

The Use of Operant Conditioning in the Investigation of Behavioral Thermoregulation

Studies such as those cited above demonstrate the effectiveness of behavior in the regulation of body temperature and draw attention to the existence of preferred temperatures. The investigation of behavioral temperature regulation has now been taken a step further by experiments employing the technique of operant conditioning. In operant conditioning, the experimenter arranges that a given action on the part of the animal be followed by a particular event. The action made by the animal is termed the "response" and can be any action chosen by the experimenter, but it is convenient to select an action, such as pressing a lever, that can be made to close a switch. The event that follows the response is said to be "positive reinforcement" if the frequency with which the animal makes the response increases. For example, a hungry animal soon learns to operate a lever when the reinforcement is a small quantity of food. This basic situation has many variations and in some studies the animal may have to make the response several times before the reinforcement is

Measuring the Demand for Heat by Operant Conditioning

In the first experiments by Carlton and Marks (1958) and Weiss and Laties (1961), rats from which the fur had been shaved learned to make a response for either a puff of warm air or a short burst of infrared heat. The animals, however, proved rather difficult to train and it was concluded that subcutaneous temperatures had to fall before regular reinforcements were obtained, although once the animal was trained it began to respond for heat as soon as it was placed in a cold ambient temperature.

Similar experiments have been done by several workers, and although it has been found that rats with fur do respond for heat they are trained only with great difficulty, and it is more usual to use shaved animals. These studies on rats have since been extended and similar experiments have been made on mice (Baldwin, 1968), monkeys (Carlisle, 1966a), and pigs (Baldwin and Ingram, 1967). It has been established that the number of reinforcements obtained per unit time increases linearly as the ambient temperature declines. A complication that arises in this respect is that at low temperatures pigs may spend time trying to escape from the cage and hence the number of reinforcements obtained declines. At any given ambient temperature, the number of reinforcements obtained per unit time depends on both the duration and the intensity of the heating.

The pig can also learn to operate a switch that turns off a fan for a short interval. Again, in this situation, it is found that the number of responses made increases as ambient temperature declines. At environmental temperatures above the critical temperature for a pig in an ambient of high air movement, very few responses are made. It appears to make little difference whether the animal is making a response for extra heat or avoiding a convective heat loss. The reinforcement value falls almost to nil within the thermoneutral zone.

When operant conditioning was first used to investigate behavior in relation to thermoregulation, the experiments always involved reinforcement with heat in a cold environment. Subsequently, studies were made in which the animal was able to escape from a heat stress, for example, by turning off a heater (Lipton, 1971), or by making a response when the reinforcement was a puff of cool air (Murgatroyd and Hardy, 1970) or a shower of water (Epstein and Milestone, 1968). It was found that rats responded for cold air reinforcement as soon as ambient temperature increased above that at which it had been found, in other experiments, that heat was no longer reinforcing. Ambient temperature had to increase much more (to 32–33°C) before animals would make a response for a shower of water. These differences in the ambient temperature at which different types of cooling became reinforcing reflected the fact that evaporative cooling in the form of licking the fur was not employed by rats unless the heat stress was fairly severe. In experiments using either form of cooling, the responses, once they had been initiated, increased linearly as ambient temperature increased, at least during short experimental sessions.

Control of Thermoregulatory Behavior

The first experiments on the possible role of deep body temperature receptors in the control of behavioral temperature regulation were made by Satinoff (1964). She trained rats to make a response for a reinforcement of infrared heat and demonstrated that if the hypothalamic region of the brain was cooled by an implanted thermode, then the animals would make responses even in a thermoneutral environment. Later, Baldwin and Ingram (1968) confirmed the effects of cooling the hypothalamus in the pig and showed that the number of responses made while the hypothalamus was held at a given temperature depended on the ambient temperature. Heating the hypothalamus decreased the response rate in the cold. In a hot environment cooling the hypothalamus was sometimes without effect. Similar effects have also been reported for monkeys and baboons (Adair et al., 1970; Gale et al., 1970) and the rat (Carlisle, 1966b).

In addition, it is now known that heating the hypothalamus increases the response rate for a reinforcement of cool air in a hot environment, whereas cooling it decreases the rate. The interaction of central and peripheral thermal stimulation on the rat's rate of responding for both heating and cooling has been studied by Murgatroyd and Hardy (1970). Using the apparatus illustrated in Fig. 7–8, they have confirmed previous findings that the rate at which reinforcements of heat are obtained in a cold environment increases when the hypothalamus is cooled and decreases when it is warmed. In a warm environment, however, although heating the hypothalamus always increases the rate at which responses are made for a puff of cool air, cooling the hypothalamus has relatively little effect in depressing the response rate until the ambient temperature is 41°C. Parallel studies on the monkey (Adair et al., 1970; Stitt et al., 1971) have demonstrated that when the animals can adjust the tem-

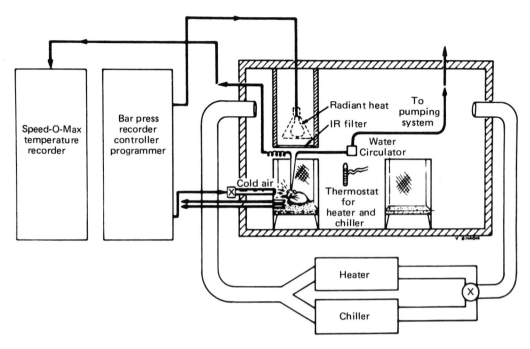

Fig. 7–8. Apparatus used to study operant behavior in a rat. Behavior can be reinforced with either infrared heat or cool air (Murgatroyd and Hardy, 1970; courtesy Charles C Thomas, publisher, Springfield, Illinois).

perature of the cage either up or down, cooling a thermode in the hypothalamus leads to an increase in ambient temperature. Heating the thermode causes the monkey to lower the cage temperature. When the thermode is heated, however, it makes no difference whether the experiment lasts 10 minutes or 2 hours, although if the thermode is cooled for 2 hours the monkey gradually allows the cage temperature to return to a neutral temperature. This apparent anomaly is possibly related to the fact that after prolonged cooling of the hypothalamus the rest of the body tends to increase in temperature and so some other thermosensitive region may have been stimulated. A similar finding has been reported by Gale et al. (1970) in the baboon. They have shown that the rate of responding during cooling of the hypothalamus falls to the control level once midbrain temperature has reached a steady level.

Findings such as these have drawn attention to the importance of thermosensitive regions outside the hypothalamus and deep in the body core. In this connection, Lipton (1971) has advanced evidence suggesting that the medulla of the rat may be one such region. Thauer (1970) has drawn attention to the role of the spinal cord in mammals and in the pigeon, and Carlisle and Ingram (1973) have compared the behavioral effects of changing the spinal temperature with changing the hypothalamic temperature in the pig.

There is a further point in connection with a changing temperature of the hypothalamus. As Corbit (1970) has pointed out, when the hypothalamus is heated there is a tendency for blood flow to the skin to increase and so raise skin temperature; cooling the hypothalamus has the opposite effect. It is therefore possible that the effects attributed to central stimuli may in some instances be related to peripheral temperature changes consequent on the central stimulus. Under some conditions, the vasomotor effects of changing hypothalamic temperature cannot be eliminated. In pigs exposed to low temperatures, however, it is known that vasoconstriction is almost complete and cooling the hypothalamus can therefore cause no further vasoconstriction. Nevertheless, cooling the hypothalamus in a cold environment leads to a marked increase in the response rate for heat reinforcement. Moreover, Satinoff (1964) and Carlisle (1966b) have measured skin temperature and have not found changes that explain the modification in response rate. It therefore seems unlikely that the whole effect of temperature changes in the hypothalamus can be related to the consequent temperature changes at the periphery, although the possibility that there is a contribution under some circumstances cannot be eliminated.

The point that emerges from these studies is that behavioral thermoregulation is influenced by temperature changes at various places, all over the body. At present, our knowledge of the distribution of these thermosensitive regions and their relative importance is incomplete.

Temperature Sensation in Man

In man, it is possible not only to assess the temperature that is selected but also to make subjective assessments about the acceptability of a given temperature. From a number of studies, it is evident that, provided the body temperature is within the normal range, the mean skin temperature is closely correlated with subjective assessments of comfort. Hardy (1971) has analyzed the results obtained by a number of workers for both clothed and nude subjects. He has concluded that at skin temperatures between 32°C and 35°C there is very little sensation of either warmth or cold; the maximum degree of comfort is reported at about 33°C. Over this 3°C range of temperature, there are nevertheless considerable changes in heat loss.

These skin temperatures, of course, do not define any particular environmental temperature because they can be produced by a variety of conditions that depend on a number of variables, such as humidity, air movement, radiant heat load, and insulation provided by clothing. Such findings suggest that behavioral reactions to ambient conditions in man may depend on skin temperature alone, but other studies have demonstrated that subjective feelings about skin temperature can be modified by changes in core temperature.

In some experiments by Cabanac (1969), subjects were placed in a water bath up to the chin. They were then asked to dip one hand into a separate test bath and to say whether the temperature of the test water was pleasant or unpleasant. Cabanac found that although the temperature of the water bath in which the subject sat, which controlled the mean skin temperature, did not influence the subjective assessment of the test bath, the body core temperature did. For example, during hyperthermia, water at 10°C was pleasant; when the subject was hypothermic, however, 10°C water was unpleasant. Conversely, a hypothermic subject reported test water at 40°C to be pleasant, whereas a hyperthermic man found it unpleasant (Fig. 7–9).

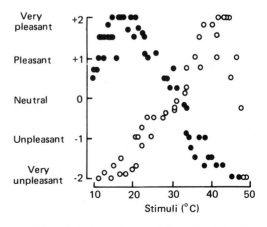

Fig. 7–9. Reactions of hypothermic (O) and hyperthermic (●) human subjects to placing the hand in water at various stimulation temperatures (Cabanac, 1969).

Benzinger (1971) considers that in the conscious sensation of bodily heat core temperature is by far the more important, because when subjects are placed in a water bath at 38°C they do not experience any sensations of alarm or discomfort until deep body temperature begins to rise. According to Benzinger, the skin is of greater importance in the detection of cold.

Lower Vertebrates

Whatever degrees of importance are attached to the central and peripheral signals, it is clear that both are involved to some degree in a wide variety of mammals. Rather less attention has been paid to the lower vertebrates, but the evidence available from studies employing operant conditioning and temperature selection demonstrates that they are able to exercise some control over the effect of the ambient conditions. Rozin and Meyer (1961) have subjected goldfish to a heat stress and then trained them to perform a response consisting of swimming against a ring for reinforcement with a jet of cold water. In the absence of the cool jets of water, the aquarium temperature increases to near the lethal limit of 41°C, but the fish maintain the temperature between 33°C and 36.5°C. In these studies, however, the fish appear to have been avoiding a heat stress rather than selecting an optimal temperature, because in thermocline experiments the same species chooses water at 25°–27°C. In the much larger arctic sculpin fish, Stromme et al. (1971) have implanted thermodes into the brain rostral to the optic chiasma. They have found that cooling the thermode causes the fish to remain in warm water for longer periods than in control experiments. In some instances, the fish have had to be removed in order to avoid the possibility of overheating.

Lizards have been studied in shuttle boxes, where they can move between two temperatures (Cabanac and Hammel, 1971), and it has been found that the movements depend on a number of factors. A rapid change in temperature is effective in causing the animal to move, but a slow change is ignored. It has also been found that the animals tolerate a low temperature for longer if the chamber is dark. Using a different procedure, Regal (1971) has found that the presence of another lizard influences the selected temperature. He has trained animals to mount a platform and to press down on a lever that keeps an infrared heater going. When a pair of lizards are placed in the cage, the dominant member spends more time obtaining heat than when it is alone.

These behavioral patterns, again, appear to be controlled by both peripheral and central temperatures. Myhre and Hammel (1969) have found that the colonic temperature at which a lizard leaves the hot part of the shuttle box decreases as the ambient temperature increases, which suggests the importance of peripheral rather than central receptors. In the same series of experiments, however, it has been found that if the brain stem is cooled by means of a thermode then the colonic temperature at which the lizards leave the test chamber increases. Warming the brainstem decreases the colonic temperature at which the lizards escape.

The control of behavioral thermoregulation therefore appears to involve a number of factors common to vertebrates as a whole. In the mammals, control depends on thermal signals that are similar to those involved in other means of thermoregulation. Corbit (1970) has suggested that models similar to those used to describe thermoregulation by vasomotor changes and evaporative heat loss may also be appropriate for behavioral thermoregulation.

CHAPTER 8

Thermosensitivity and the Thermoregulatory System

The integrated response of a mammal to heat stress must obviously depend on a complex regulatory system. In chapters 4, 5, 6, and 7, various experiments have been described that have involved warming the whole animal or heating part of its peripheral or core tissue locally. These have provided abundant evidence that thermoregulation depends on stimuli received at many sites. The information received at these sites must then be compared and processed in some center or centers where decisions are made and instructions sent out to the various effector mechanisms (see Hensel, 1973, for a review of the neural processes involved). In this chapter, the sites of these regulatory centers are considered and the thermosensitive elements on which the regulatory system is based are discussed. Finally, some attention is given to the various types of models that have been proposed to describe the thermoregulatory system.

Central Thermosensitive Cells

The Hypothalamus

The significance of the hypothalamus as a region not only sensitive to changes in local temperature but also containing cells that play an important part in the control of body temperature has been recognized for over a hundred years. The very considerable numbers of experiments involving local heating or cooling, electrical stimulation, and the placement of discrete lesions have been reviewed by Bligh (1966, 1973) and only the main conclusions of these studies are mentioned here. From a number of experiments involving the placement of lesions (e.g., Ranson and Ingram, 1935; Ranson and Magoun, 1939), it has been shown that if the preoptic region of the hypothalamus is destroyed the animal is unable to regulate its body temperature properly in a hot environment but may still be able to thermoregulate on exposure to cold. Destruction of the posterior region of the hypothalamus that also destroys fibers passing up to the preoptic region, however, leads to loss of the ability to thermoregulate in hot and cold environments.

These findings have been used as evidence to support the hypothesis, first advanced by Meyer (1913), that there are two centers in the hypothalamus that control thermoregulation; one in the anterior region, which is thermolytic, and the other in the posterior region, which is thermogenic. The idea is an attractive one and is to some extent supported by observations on humans with brain tumors that have destroyed parts of the hypothalamus. Moreover, electrical stimulation of the anterior hypothalamus (Andersson et al., 1956) causes vasodilatation and panting and also inhibits shivering, whereas stimulation of several places in the midbrain has been shown to cause shivering and vasoconstriction.

The simple concept of two anatomically discrete antagonistic centers, however, does not explain all the well-established observations on the temperature sensitivity of the hypothalamus. It has been shown, for example, that cooling the preoptic region elicits a rise in metabolic rate and behavioral responses appropriate to cold exposure. It has also been shown that there are neurons in the preoptic region that increase their rates of firing when the local temperature falls. There appears, therefore, to be no clearcut spatial separation of the neuronal elements concerned with heat loss and heat conservation.

Even after the hypothalamus has been destroyed, some ability to regulate body temperature may persist. For example, Andersson et al. (1965) have found that animals with lesions in the hypothalamus may still respond to a hot environment by panting, but only after body temperature has increased to over 41°C. The possibility discussed by Bligh (1966) is that other regulatory "centers" also influence heat loss, although they lack the fine control exercised by the hypothalamus.

The Spinal Cord

The local thermosensitivity of the spinal cord has been discovered much more recently than that of the hypothalamus but has nevertheless stimulated a great deal of study (see reviews by Thauer, 1970; Klussmann and Pierau, 1972). Heating and cooling the cord is accompanied by responses similar to those observed on heating and cooling the hypothalamus. The effects of changing the cord temperature can be reduced by changing the hypothalamic temperature in the opposite direction, or enhanced when hypothalamic temperature is changed in the same direction, as that of the cord. The thermosensitive elements involved in these reactions are located within the cord itself and some of the effects of local temperature changes can still be observed when the cord is isolated from the brain. Even in a dog in which the spinal cord has been cut, for example, changes in skin blood flow and shivering can still be elicited by changing the temperature of the cord locally. At least part of the ability of animals with hypothalamic lesions to achieve some control over body temperature may therefore depend on the activity of the spinal cord.

An observation rather more difficult to explain is that some animals may still display some degree of thermoregulation even after the spinal cord has been destroyed, cutting off the neural connections of the hypothalamus from the effector mechanisms, such as shivering. In such animals, however, the intact hypothalamus still controls hormonal activity and it has been suggested that this may explain the residual thermoregulatory capacity provided body temperature is allowed to shift far enough to activate the hypothalamus in the absence of information from the periphery.

Thermosensitivity of Other Regions

Although some responses have been observed after changing the temperature of the medulla locally, their significance to thermoregulation is not clear. In some animals, heating and cooling the abdomen has been observed to activate thermoregulatory mechanisms, suggesting a concentration of thermosensitive cells in this region. It has also been suggested that the walls of the great veins contain thermosensitive cells, or that the sensors may also be located in muscle fibers. As far as is known, these cells probably feed their information into the control center in the same way as do the thermoreceptors in the skin.

Peripheral Thermosensitive Cells

The existence of thermosensitivity to both heat and cold in the skin is a matter of common experience, as is the existence of temperature receptors on the tongue. The importance of these receptors has been demonstrated by experiments in which changes in skin temperature have elicited a thermoregulatory response in the absence of any change in core temperature.

Thermosensitive Cells and Thermoreceptors

Almost all cells in the nervous system are influenced by temperature, as are the various metabolic processes that occur in cells throughout the body. The changes in the activity of biological reactions with temperature usually have a Q_{10} of about $+2$ and can be explained on the basis of the Arrhenius-Van't Hoff effect, which describes how most chemical reactions proceed faster at higher temperatures. It is in spite of this effect of temperature that animal systems have evolved for regulating body temperature about a fairly constant value and have developed nervous mechanisms that can estimate temperature.

Just how biological systems either maintain a standard reference point for temperature or achieve thermostability and measure temperature without one is not understood. Some of the elements on which the system is most likely to depend have been identified. These consist of some cells that are particularly sensitive to changes in temperature and others that are remarkable for the absence of temperature dependence. Temperature-sensitive cells are usually described as "cold sensitive" if their activity increases with a fall in temperature and as "warm sensitive" if it increases with a rise in temperature. However, this division does not necessarily mean that the cold-sensitive neurons are concerned solely with defense against a cold ambient and *vice versa*. The cold thermoreceptors, in fact, are still active at temperatures that are considered warm. Moreover, it is obvious that a neuron which decreases its activity as temperature increases can just as readily be used to control heat loss mechanisms as one which increases activity with a rise in temperature.

Temperature Receptors

The identification of the morphological features that characterize temperature receptors has been an intractable task. The original idea, that the Krause endings are cold receptors and the Ruffini endings are warm receptors, has proved to be false. One difficulty is that temperature influences sensory endings in general and mechanoreceptors are particularly sensitive. As an aid to elucidating the problem Hensel et al. (1960) have suggested a number of properties that should be displayed by specific thermorecep-tors. These are: (1) the sensitivity should not change when the temperature is held constant. (2) Specific thermoreceptors should have a dynamic sensitivity to changes in tem-perature with a temperature coefficient that is positive for warm receptors and negative for cold receptors. (3) They should not readily be excited by mechanical and other nonthermal stimulation. (4) Their threshold sensitivity should be similar to perceptual thermal thresholds where it is possible to test the point.

The species that have received most at-tention are man, cat, dog, rat, and monkey. Cold-sensitive endings, possibly simply be-cause they are more numerous, have been studied more often than those responsive to warmth. Both types of receptor appear un-der the light microscope as "free" nerve end-ings, which is only to say that their special-ized structure is too small to be seen. Very little is known about the actual transducer mechanisms by which temperature is used to produce a generator potential. Most prob-ably, the mechanism depends on such param-eters as membrane resistance and potas-sium conductance, which vary according to the temperature. These in turn may be re-lated to changes in the structure of the mem-brane, such as the melting transition from the crystalline to the liquid state of certain phospholipids, or the change from a crys-talline to an amorphous state by certain proteins (Sperelakis, 1970). It is at least plausible that variations in the type of phos-pholipid and protein of the membrane of receptors account for the differences that have been observed with respect to the tem-perature at which the peak sensitivity of a receptor occurs.

Most of the information about temper-ature receptors is derived from studies of impulses propagated along the nerve fiber when the receptor is stimulated by means of a fine-pointed thermode. In the cat, dog, and rat, the thermoreceptors on the general body surface of the trunk and limbs have nonmye-linated C fibers. Thermoreceptors with mye-linated A fibers do occur in the mouth and nose of cats and dogs, however, and on the body surface of primates.

When the temperature over the receptor is kept constant, the rate of discharge along the fiber is also constant and remains so over many hours of recording. At some other temperature a new rate of discharge is estab-lished and is again maintained for as long as the temperature is constant. From experi-ments of this kind, graphs of discharge rate against temperature have been constructed. These reveal the range of temperatures over which the receptor is responsive and the tem-perature at which maximum sensitivity oc-curs. Such curves describe the static sensi-tivity of the receptor.

Two families of receptor can be de-tected by this method: the "cold" receptors, which are active over a fairly wide range of about 5°–43°C and have maxima between 20°C and 35°C (Hensel, 1970), and the "warm" receptors, which begin to discharge at close to 35°C and have a maximum dis-charge rate at 43°–45°C, above which re-sponse falls off rapidly. Figure 8–1 shows graphs for the two kinds of receptor. An im-portant additional distinction between the two types of receptors can be made with re-spect to their response to a change in tem-perature; that is, they have distinctive dy-namic sensitivities. If the temperature of a cold receptor is allowed to fall, there is an initial burst of activity, which then declines.

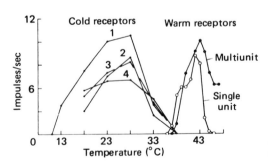

Fig. 8–1. Response of "warm" and "cold" peripheral temperature receptors (Iggo, 1969).

In contrast, a rise in temperature is accompanied by a temporary inhibition of nervous discharge. Warm receptors behave in the opposite manner, with a burst of activity when temperature rises and inhibition when it falls. A second graph can therefore be constructed for each receptor, relating discharge rate to temperature immediately after the temperature is changed and describing its dynamic sensitivity.

As has been shown by Iggo (1969), the two types of sensitivity, static and dynamic, are related because the increase in discharge rate when temperature is changed is a constant proportion of the resting discharge rate (Fig. 8–2). In the monkey, mye-

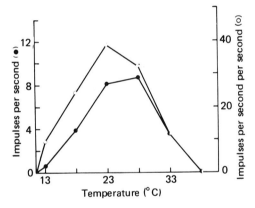

Fig. 8–2. The "static" (●—●) and "dynamic" (○—○) response curves of thermoreceptors (Iggo, 1969).

linated fibers from cold receptors in the skin have been found from which recordings with an additional property have been made. In these fibers, the discharge occurs in bursts when the temperature of the receptor is at or near the temperature of maximum sensitivity and then becomes more continuous at higher temperature. Iggo (1969) has pointed out that this phenomenon may be of advantage in distinguishing between a possible ambiguity in the information provided by the receptor. For example, in Fig. 8–1 it can be seen that in the rat the same discharge rate

is associated with two widely different temperatures, and additional information may be provided by the bursts of activity in the monkey's receptors.

A further set of receptors has been found that does not begin to respond until the temperature is above 46°C. Some cold receptors in the tongue, moreover, become active again at high temperatures. The value of these thermoreceptors is not clear, but they may serve in some way to protect the animal against dangerously high temperatures.

The nerve fibers described so far are specifically sensitive to heat and are not easily activated by mechanical stimuli to the receptor. Some fibers have been found, however, that belong to receptors with a low threshold to mechanical stimulation and that nevertheless respond to changes in temperature in a manner similar to cold receptors. Such fibers have a steady rate of firing when the receptor is at a constant temperature, increase the rate of firing when the temperature falls, and are inhibited when temperature rises. They differ from "true" cold receptors in having a monotonic response, with a high discharge rate at low temperatures that declines steadily as temperature rises to 40°C and higher. The significance to thermoregulation of the thermosensitivity of these receptors is not clear, for although they respond to temperature changes, the central nervous system may not be able to differentiate between discharges related to mechanical and to thermal stimuli.

The next problem that must be discussed is the surface area served by a single fiber and the exact nature of the thermal stimulus that initiates discharge along a fiber. Using a very fine-pointed thermode placed on the skin or surface of the tongue, Hensel (1970) has found that the receptive area for some fibers is a point 1 or 2 mm in diameter, but other fibers may be affected by temperature changes in a receptive area up to 1.7 cm². This finding fits in with studies on man, which have suggested that the skin has discrete spots that are sensitive to temperature.

Experiments regarding the exact nature of the thermal stimulus have been reviewed by Hensel (1963, 1970). One investigated possibility is that the receptors are not actually sensitive to temperature *per se* but only to slight fluctuations in temperature. Even in very carefully controlled studies it is difficult to eliminate the possibility of small changes in the temperature of the thermode stimulating the receptor. The experiment in which this idea has been tested has therefore been made on cold receptors during slight ($0.05°C$/second) but continuous warming. With this rate of warming no inhibition occurs, but the rate of discharge along the fiber declines. Moreover, a fall of $0.1°C$/second is accompanied by an even greater fall in the frequency of discharge without any inhibition. A corresponding result is obtained with warm receptors exposed to slow cooling and it is concluded that the receptors are in fact sensitive to temperature as such.

A second idea is that as the receptors are known usually to be arborized, the real stimulus might in fact be a small thermal gradient across the receptor terminals. This hypothesis has been tested by Hensel and Witt (1959) with the receptors in the cat's tongue. In this study, the tongue was placed between two thermodes and a fiber associated with a single "cool" spot on the upper surface was dissected out. The upper surface of the tongue was then held at a lower temperature than the under side and a recording of the discharge rate along the fiber was made. One thermode on the under surface was then cooled, with the results that (1) the gradient across the tongue was reversed and (2) the temperature of the whole tongue, including its upper surface, began to fall. The discharge rate along the fiber increased steadily during this procedure. If the receptor had been sensitive to a temperature gradient, then the discharge would have been expected to stop. Temperature receptors, therefore, or at least those in the cat's

tongue, do not depend on a temperature gradient across the terminals.

Central Effects of Peripheral Thermal Stimulation

The results so far described have related to recordings obtained from presynaptic nerve fibers close to the receptor site. It is also possible to detect the effects of stimulating peripheral receptors by recording from cells in the thalamus and the sensory cortex. Some of the neurons in the cat's cortex respond to heating, cooling, and tactile stimulation of the tongue. These nonspecific effects may be related to stimulation of mechanoreceptors or may be the result of synaptic convergence. In either event, their significance to thermoregulation is not clear.

Some neurons in the cortex and the thalamus, however, respond only to cooling of a specific spot on the tongue and are quite unaffected by chemical and tactile stimulation. Neurons that respond only to warming the tongue are rather less numerous than those that respond to cooling, but they are also unaffected by other stimuli (Landgren, 1970). Projections on to the cortex have also been demonstrated for warm receptors on the scrotum (Hellon and Provins, 1972). Some of the cortical cells are inhibited from firing when the scrotum is warmed and others increased their firing rate, but neither type of cell responds when the scrotum is subjected to nonthermal stimulation.

What is not known at present is whether the same receptor in the skin has projections that influence both the conscious perception of temperature and the autonomic thermoregulatory system. From what is known of the central nervous system in general, however, it should not be surprising to find that the same receptor serves both functions.

Thermosensitive Neurons in the Hypothalamus

The discovery of units in the hypothalamus that display a marked response in the discharge rate with change in temperature is a relatively recent event. Because it has not been possible to demonstrate unequivocally that the units from which recordings have been made are true thermoreceptors, comparable to those in the skin, they are referred to here simply as "thermosensitive." The technique used in these studies involves implanting microelectrodes and thermodes into the hypothalamus and changing the temperature locally while recording the firing rate of individual units. Even after contact has been established with a given cell, however, the only way of telling whether it is temperature sensitive is to change the temperature and record the response. Consequently, a large number of units may be examined, only a few of which prove to be thermosensitive. Moreover, once found, the technical difficulties of maintaining contact are such that a unit may be lost before all the required information has been obtained.

In the first study of this kind, by Nakayama et al. (1961) on anesthetized animals, no cold-sensitive neurons that increased their rate of firing when the temperature fell were found. However, neurons that increased their rate of firing with an increase in temperature were demonstrated.

Since then, a considerable number of studies have been made (see reviews by Hellon, 1970; Eisenman, 1972) and several kinds of units with probable importance in thermoregulation have been described in conscious and anesthetized animals. Most of the neurons that have been described as thermosensitive increase their rate of firing as temperature increases over the normal range of core temperature (warm sensitive). However, a few units in the preoptic region have also been found that increase their firing rate as temperature falls (cold sensitive).

These straight-line relations between temperature and firing rate, first discovered using small temperature ranges, have since been reexamined over much wider temperature ranges (Cabanac et al., 1968). Under these conditions, the relations between discharge frequency and temperature take the form of bell-shaped curves, not unlike those obtained for peripheral thermoreceptors. They are illustrated diagramatically in Fig. 8–3A and B.

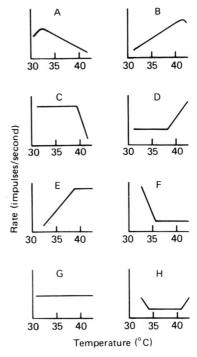

Fig. 8–3. Diagrammatic representation of the responses of various neurons in the hypothalamus to local changes in temperature.

A difficulty that arises with units deep in the central nervous system is that they may be influenced synaptically by other neurons. The problem is therefore to decide whether the unit from which a recording is being taken is itself thermosensitive, or whether it is being driven synaptically by some other thermoreceptor. In order to investigate this matter further, the effect of anesthetics on the frequency of firing has been studied. Because barbiturates act by blocking synaptic transmission, and because they have very little influence on the type of neuron described above, these neurons may indeed be primary thermosensitive cells. They occur throughout the hypothalamus but are much more numerous in the preoptic region than in the posterior zone.

Another group of neurons in the hypothalamus, displaying a biphasic relation between temperature and firing rate, has also been described. Because these are particularly sensitive to barbiturates, they have been regarded as interneurons that are driven synaptically. Throughout the hypothalamus, the shape of the biphasic relation of firing rate and temperature falls very broadly into four groups, illustrated in a highly idealized form in Fig. 8–3C, D, E, and F. In each instance the unit displays almost no change in firing rate over some part of the temperature range, but then, at some point, the firing rate either increases or decreases abruptly.

A particularly interesting group of neurons appears to be completely insensitive to temperature; that is, these neurons do not even display the Q_{10} of 2 that is to be expected of biological systems (Fig. 8–3G). Just what sort of mechanism compensates for temperature so nicely in these cells is not known, but it is neurons of this kind that may act as reference points against which temperature can be judged.

Last, Eisenman (1972), has found a unit in the posterior hypothalamus that operates only at the extreme ranges of temperature and responds with an increased discharge to both very warm and very cool temperatures (Fig. 8–3H).

The influence of thermal stimulation of the skin on units in the preoptic hypothalamus was first demonstrated by Wit and Wang (1968). They found some units that responded to heating of the skin with an unexplained delay of 2–5 minutes after the application of the stimulus, but nevertheless before brain temperature changed. When the local temperature did increase, however,

there was a further increase in firing rate. Hellon (1970) found units in the preoptic region that responded to cooling the skin with an increase in firing rate, as well as those that responded to heating. In addition, some units responded to both local and peripheral temperature, indicating a convergence of pathways.

As expected from studies involving warming and cooling of both the spine and the hypothalamus, it has also been possible to demonstrate units in the preoptic region that are inhibited when the spine is heated (Guieu and Hardy, 1970b). There is also evidence of convergence of pathways, for some units respond both to local changes of temperature in the hypothalamus and to changes in cord temperature.

The occurrence of units in the hypothalamus that respond both to local temperature changes and to changes in temperature elsewhere illustrates the very complex nature of the interconnections. It also underlines the difficulty of distinguishing between primary and secondary thermosensitivity.

Thermosensitivity of Units Outside the Hypothalamus

Further back in the midbrain reticular formation, Nakayama and Hardy (1969) have found units that give a linear response to local cooling and also respond to local cooling or mechanical stimulation of the skin. Some units in the preoptic region of the hypothalamus respond to cooling of the midbrain but no midbrain units have been found that respond to changes in the temperature of the preoptic zone. In other words, the convergence of information seems to be directed toward the hypothalamus in particular. Within the spinal cord itself, Wünnerberg and Brück (1968) and Simon and Iriki (1971) have found units in the afferent pathway to the brain that increase their firing rate when the temperature of the cord is changed, although definite primary thermosensors have not been identified.

The observation that animals with severed spinal cords can shiver in response to local cooling of the spine has led to the investigation of the local thermal sensitivity of the efferent neurons that may be involved in this mechanism. Recordings made from motoneurons indicate that these units are themselves thermosensitive and increase their firing rate when cooled. Klussmann and Pierau (1972) have reviewed the experiments published on this point. They suggest that when the motoneuron is cooled it becomes more excitable and so responds more readily to incoming excitatory impulses. The synaptic connections onto these motoneurons, they suggest, include inputs from the periphery, those from thermosensors in the cord, and descending fibers from the brain.

Neuron Models of Thermoregulation

The identification of several types of thermosensitive and insensitive neurons, some of which are much better documented than others, has naturally led to speculation about the role played by the various units in the control system. Bligh (1972) has reviewed the literature that has accumulated on this subject and has illustrated some of the proposed neuron networks. All the models are necessarily much simpler than the actual system is likely to be, and all are highly speculative. Moreover, as this aspect of thermoregulation is relatively new, we almost certainly have not yet identified all the elements involved, and even some of those that have been identified have only been demonstrated once. A note of caution is also sounded by the discoveries of thermosensitive units in the sensory cortex and of some thermosensitive motoneurons (Klussmann

and Pierau, 1972) that may have very little if anything to do with thermoregulation. Current neuronal models are therefore likely to be modified in the near future and, for this reason, their various merits are not discussed in detail here. The principles on which the models are based are more likely to stand the test of time, however, and some consideration is given to them.

The evidence for the existence of true thermoreceptors at the periphery is fairly complete, but it is also explicitly assumed by those constructing neuronal models that the central "warm"- and "cold"-sensitive neurons are also primary thermoreceptors in the same sense. There is evidence that the information from various receptors converges in the hypothalamus and also good reason to believe that most of the decisions are taken here. The hypothalamus is therefore likely to contain some mechanism corresponding to a set-point temperature; when this is exceeded, heat loss mechanisms are stimulated and heat conservation is inhibited.

Some possible ways this may be achieved are illustrated in Fig. 8–4. In this network, the set point is determined by the crossover point of a "warm"- and a "cold"-sensitive unit. If the outputs of these units are fed onto the same interneuron, then this interneuron exhibits the characteristics of one of the thermosensitive interneurons that have been described above. This model also involves a neuron that changes the sign of the impulse from the warm sensor on its way to the heat conservation mechanism and so inhibits conservation as temperature rises. Such a sign-reversing interneuron also gives a linear response to temperature change but may be expected to be sensitive to anesthetics. As long as the temperature is below the set point, the inhibitory impulses from the cold sensor on the heat loss neuron exceed the excitatory ones from the warm sensor and the unit does not discharge. Above the set point, the unit begins to discharge and its firing rate increases with temperature.

A very similar arrangement can be constructed using a temperature-insensitive neuron and a warm sensor (Fig. 8–5). The combination of both suggested networks, in Fig. 8–6, provides for vasomotor tone to be decreased at a lower temperature than that at which evaporative heat loss is increased. The temperature-insensitive neuron is used to inhibit evaporative heat loss until a higher temperature has been reached. The network indicates that only the "warm" sensor on the temperature-insensitive neuron influences vasomotor tone, but clearly it may be modified to include an input from the "cold" sensor as well. However, the demonstration that the units that are known to exist can function to provide a "set point" should not be taken as proof that a reference signal is used as a "set point." As discussed below, it is possible to construct a model that depends on a dynamic control.

These models involve only one set of temperature sensors. A network that can begin to explain all the influences that are

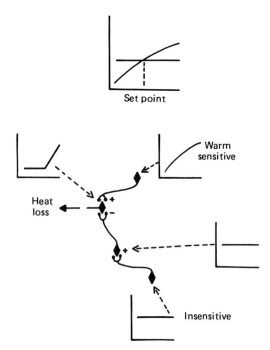

Fig. 8–5. Another possible arrangement of neurons that could provide a set point temperature reference using a "warm"-sensitive and an "insensitive" cell.

already known must at least include inputs from thermoreceptors in the skin and the spinal cord and may also involve others. In addition, nonthermal stimuli must also be included because these obviously influence such mechanisms as vasomotor tone and respiratory frequency. The difficulty with such models is that they are likely to become so complicated that they limit their own usefulness as aids to understanding the mechanism they seek to explain.

Local Injections into the Lateral Ventricles and the Hypothalamus

Pyrogens

A technique that has proved of particular value in understanding the thermoregulatory mechanism has involved the local

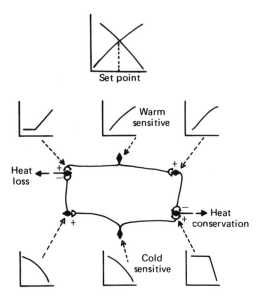

Fig. 8–4. A possible arrangement of neurons that could provide a set point temperature reference using a "cold"- and a "warm"-sensitive cell. The response characteristics of each neuron involved is indicated: (+) indicates stimulation, (−) indicates inhibition at the synapse.

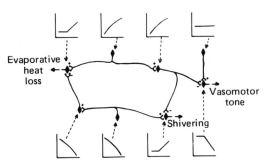

Fig. 8–6. A very simple arrangement of neurons that could provide for the control of body temperature. The warm-sensitive primary thermosensitive neuron in the upper row feeds on to a cell on the left, which is also influenced by the cold-sensitive primary thermosensitive cell in the bottom row. Evaporative heat loss is thus provided with a control using the system shown in Fig. 8–4. The warm-sensitive neuron also controls vasomotor tone through a system similar to that shown in Fig. 8–5, but the temperature ranges over which evaporative heat loss and vasomotor tone are varied can be different. Shivering is controlled by the same system as the evaporative heat loss and in this model shivering starts when evaporative loss stops.

injection of substances into the lateral ventricles of the brain, or directly into the hypothalamus or the third ventricle. This technique has led to interesting results with respect to pyrogens (Eisenman, 1972). When these substances are injected while recordings are being made from a warm-sensitive neuron, it is found that there is a decrease in the slope of the line relating firing rate to temperature. As can be seen by reference to Figs. 8–4 or 8–5 this must result in raising the set point and allowing body temperature to rise, which is, of course, just what happens in fever.

Transmitter Substance

The technique of intraventricular injections has also given rise to a considerable literature on the effects of neurotransmitter substances. The injection of a transmitter substance into the cerebral ventricles may have been expected to lead to a confused assortment of reactions as various neural pathways are activated. In fact, Feldberg and Myers (1964) have observed an apparently well-integrated response of the thermoregulatory system in the cat when they have injected 5-hydroxytryptamine (5-HT) or catecholamines. After treatment with noradrenaline or adrenaline, rectal temperature declines for an hour or two but after the injection of 5-HT, rectal temperature increases and remains high for more than 12 hours.

The effects of transmitter substances have now been examined in a number of animals (see review by Hellon, 1970) and a surprising species difference in response has emerged. In the cat, dog, and monkey, noradrenaline increases temperature and 5-HT depresses it, whereas in the sheep and rabbit the effect is just the opposite. In some other species, for example, the rat, the effect of noradrenaline appears to depend on the dose used, but the differences in response between the cat, dog, and monkey, on the one hand, and the sheep and rabbit, on the other, are not related to dose and are, it seems, genuine species differences.

An important factor in determining the animal's response to the injection of transmitter substances is the ambient temperature. For example, in the ox (Findlay and Thompson, 1968) and the cat, noradrenaline causes a fall in temperature in a cold ambient temperature, but it has no effect at warm ambients because the heat loss mechanisms are already activated. The effects of ambient temperature on the response to transmitter substances have been taken a step further by Bligh et al. (1971), working on sheep, goats, and rabbits. They have found that in a hot ambient, noradrenaline decreases panting and leads to an increase in body temperature, whereas in a cold environment, noradrenaline decreases shivering and leads to a fall in body temperature. This result is interpreted to mean that noradrenaline inhibits thermoregulatory activity in both the heat loss and the heat conservation pathways. In these species, 5-HT behaves as an excitatory transmitter acting along the heat loss pathway. It increases panting in a warm environment, with a resultant fall in body temperature, and also reduces shivering in a cold environment, also leading to a fall in body temperature.

Acetylcholine, which is well established as a peripheral transmitter substance, has been found to produce a complex response. On balance, however, it appears to be in the heat production pathway, at least in sheep and goats. Again, however, there appear to be species differences, because in rats and mice the intraventricular injection of acetylcholine leads to hypothermia.

The perfusion of the cerebral ventricles, of course, must involve large regions of the brain and possible sites of action of the transmitter substances. More precise information can be obtained by microinjection to specific regions. In studies of this kind, it has been found that the temperature effects of noradrenaline and 5-HT are obtained on injection into the preoptic region of the anterior hypothalamus, whereas acetylcholine is effective when injected into a number of places in the midbrain. These and other studies, which have involved depleting the brain of certain transmitter substances or preventing their inactivation, have confirmed their role in temperature regulation. The best method of testing the effects of a transmitter substance on individual neurons involves the use of iontophoresis and preliminary findings using this technique do not fully confirm the findings using injection. One possibility is that injection of putative transmitter substances into the brain causes the local release of other substances such as prostaglandins. The prostaglandins occur very widely throughout the body and have been found in the hypothalamus. Prostaglandin E_1 has been shown very potent indeed in causing shivering and a rise in body temperature when injected into the third ventricle in both cats and rabbits. The possi-

bility therefore arises that the transmitter substances, 5-HT and noradrenaline, act at least in part by controlling the level of prostaglandin. This is, however, a very active field of research and a definitive statement cannot yet be made.

Inorganic Ions

Perfusion of the cerebral ventricle with a fluid containing a high proportion of sodium or calcium ions also disturbs body temperature. A high concentration of sodium ions leads to hyperthermia, whereas excess calcium produces hypothermia, both effects having a duration of half a day. Moreover, the direction of temperature change that accompanies these changes in ionic balance is the same in both cat and rabbit. The possibility therefore arises that the temperature at which the body is controlled is somehow determined by the ratio of calcium and sodium ions. Experiments on the monkey (Myers and Yaksh, 1971) have demonstrated that perfusion of the ventricle with solutions rich in one of the ions can apparently reset the body thermostat. The role of ions in determining membrane potentials is very well established. Clearly, an imbalance can be expected to influence the firing rate of neurons. The change in body temperature that occurs when the ionic balance of the hypothalamus is disturbed is therefore probably related to changes in sensitivity of the thermosensitive neurons. The significance of these findings in relation to normal temperature regulation has yet to be determined.

Cross-Perfusion Experiments

The experiments on injection into the cerebral ventricles and the hypothalamus that have been outlined so far have simply demonstrated that effects can be obtained when the normal balance of substances in the brain are disturbed. Experiments on cross-perfusion, however, demonstrate that the composition of the cerebrospinal fluid is actually changed when animals are exposed to different temperatures. In these studies (Myers, 1971), the fluid from the ventricle of one monkey has been removed and perfused into the ventricle of a second monkey. When the donor animal is exposed to heat, the recipient monkey responds with a fall in body temperature; if the donor is exposed to cold, the recipient's temperature increases. There is evidence that the perfusate from the cooled monkey contains an increased amount of 5-HT, which is expected, but there is also the possibility that prostaglandins are also involved and the method of cross-perfusion obviously contains exciting possibilities.

Models of the Control System

Biological Models

The basis on which neuronal models of the regulating system are made has already been mentioned, and it should clearly be possible to incorporate the findings from studies on the injection of transmitter substances with neuron networks. Several such models have been published, and Fig. 8–7 shows one based on the work of Bligh (1972), who has commented on the similarity between models that have been arrived at by different groups using different approaches. The role of the transmitter substances is not quite so well defined and must await the results of further studies using iontophoresis techniques.

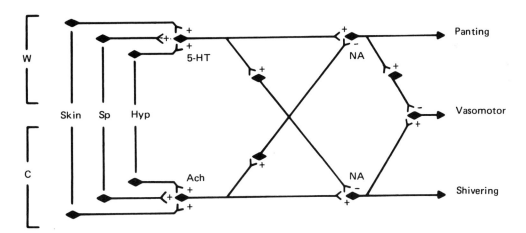

Fig. 8–7. Model of neurons in which synapses are activated by acetylcholine (Ach), 5-hydroxytryptamine (5-HT), or noradrenaline (NA). The warm (W) receptors in the skin, spinal cord, and hypothalamus all feed onto the same interneuron through a synapse that is activated by 5-HT. This neuron then activates two interneurons and inhibits shivering by one path involving NA and initiates panting by another path, also using NA. Therefore, the injection of 5-HT into the brain of an animal that is already panting in a hot environment has little effect, but in a cold environment when the animal is not panting, panting can be initiated. Noradrenaline, in contrast, inhibits panting in a hot environment and also inhibits shivering in a cold environment because it appears to be the transmitter substance involved in the cross-inhibition of warm- (W) and cold- (C) sensitive neurons. This model also provides for the control of vasomotor tone (after Bligh, 1972).

Nonbiological Models of Thermoregulation

Many physical and mathematical models have been advanced in attempts to interpret and understand information about heat exchange between animals and their environment. The subject has been discussed recently by Mitchell et al. (1972), Hardy et al. (1971), and Kerslake (1972).

Basically the mathematical model takes the form of the equation

$$\text{Heat production} = \text{heat loss}$$

This equation can be elaborated and its form may also be changed according to the particular interest on which an investigation centers e.g.:

Heat storage = heat-production − radiant heat-loss − convective heat-loss − conductive heat-loss − evaporative heat-loss

When the body is actually cooling, the heat storage term is negative. Obviously such terms as radiant heat loss in this equation can also be positive or negative, according to whether heat is being lost or gained by this channel. The equation can also be expanded to take account of evaporative heat loss, from the skin and the respiratory tract separately, and heat production can be subdivided into basal metabolism, including that associated with the work of the heart, and into shivering and nonshivering thermogenesis. Over long periods of time the importance of heat storage represented by a change in body temperature decreases, but nutritional factors become important. Heat balance equations may therefore also take the form:

Metabolizable energy intake = radiant heat loss + convective heat loss + evaporative heat loss + heat loss by conduction + energy loss in urine and feces + energy storage

In this equation, the storage term refers to energy retained as fat or protein, and any change in body temperature can be neglected.

Equations such as these simply describe the system. If after all the variables are measured they do not balance, then either there is an error in the methods of measurement, or an important variable has been omitted. For example, in an animal lying down on a cool surface, heat loss by conduction is important and failure to measure this factor and incorporate it leads to an anomalous situation. These mathematical models, however, do not reveal any information about mechanisms and they are most often employed to estimate one variable by difference when the rest have been measured directly.

As an aid to understanding thermal balance and heat-flow within the body, the mathematical model is perhaps better depicted in the form of a block diagram. In this type of model, a number of black boxes are connected by arrows and the mathematical relation between the input and output of a particular box can be indicated. A simple example of such a model is shown in Fig. 8–8, after Carlson and Hsieh (1970). Much more complex models have also been developed. Models of this kind can describe heat flow within the body, that is, the controlled system; in complex varieties the limbs, trunk, body core, and skin are separately represented and account is taken of countercurrent heat exchangers. The model itself may either be represented as a series of black boxes and transfer functions, or it takes the form of an electrical analog, in which resistance to heat flow is represented as an electrical resistance and thermal mass as a capacitance. These models are of use in predicting and understanding how heat is transferred around and from the body, but they say nothing about the controlling system.

Simple models that attempt to describe the system controlling core temperature may take the form of a mechanical analog in which the level of water in a tank is kept at a constant level in spite of disturbances to the rate at which water flows in or out.

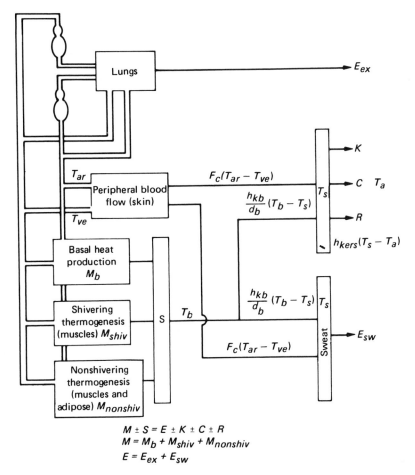

$$M \pm S = E \pm K \pm C \pm R$$
$$M = M_b + M_{shiv} + M_{nonshiv}$$
$$E = E_{ex} + E_{sw}$$

Fig. 8–8. Mathematical, black box type of model of heat conduction and convection from the interior of the body to the skin. No mechanisms are indicated but the relations between input and output of the control system are given in mathematical terms. E, total evaporative heat loss; E_{ex}, evaporative heat loss consequent on breathing; E_{sw}, evaporative heat loss consequent on sweating; M, total metabolic heat production; M_b, basal metabolic rate; M_{shiv}, heat production from shivering; $M_{nonshiv}$, heat production from nonshivering thermogenesis; S, heat storage; K, conductive heat loss; C, convective heat loss; R, radiant heat loss; F, rate of blood flow to periphery; c, specific heat of blood; T_s, skin temperature; T_b, blood temperature; h_{kcrs}, heat transfer coefficient for K, C, and R; h_{kb}, transfer coefficient for conductive heat from interior to skin; T_{ar}, temperature of blood arriving at skin $= T_b$; T_{ve}, temperature of blood leaving skin $= T_s$; d_b, distance between points at which T_b and T_s are measured (Carlson and Hsieh, 1970; by permission, copyright Loren D. Carlson).

Another form is the electrical analog, in which the maintenance of body temperature is compared with a thermostatically controlled oven. Such models as these help in forming ideas about the controlling system and can be developed by considering the various merits of on–off regulators and, say, proportional controllers, where the response of the system depends on the "load error" between the actual temperature and the "set point." Other types of regulator are the integral controller, in which response depends on both the "load error" and the time for which the actual temperature has departed from the "set point," and also rate controllers, in which the response of the controlling system depends on the rate at which the actual temperature is departing from, or coming toward, the "set point." In the final development of models of the controlling system, feedback loops must be specified and the important body temperature that is the set point must be identified.

Once the controlled and controlling systems are reasonably well understood, however, a computer can be programmed to predict what will happen in a given set of circumstances, for example, an astronaut in space, or how much exercise under given ambient conditions and clothing can be safely undertaken. Physical models using electrical heaters can also be used in practical situations as, for example, a model that indicates the heat loss of an agricultural animal when placed in a test environment, such as an animal pen.

CHAPTER 9

Animals in Hot Environments

Animal production and activity in a hot environment are particularly hampered by diminished feed intake and by the need to dissipate the additional heat associated with productivity under conditions of thermal neutrality or higher temperatures.

One of the effects of a high temperature is to diminish appetite, so that feed intake and consequently energy retention both decrease; this has led to the search for heat-adapted animals and means of enhancing adaptation to heat. Another approach to combating high temperatures is through environmental control, using shades and wallows to counteract the heating effects of the animal's surroundings. Other difficulties facing animal production in hot regions of the world are the lack of suitable forage during some seasons and the high fiber content and low protein value of much of the available forage.

The need to dissipate additional heat arises because the partial efficiency of utilization of metabolic energy for growth is less than unity and is usually about 0.6–0.7. For each increment in energy retention, then, 30–40 percent of the associated metabolizable energy must be dissipated as heat. Under cold conditions, in contrast, although the partial efficiency of the growth process is similar, the excess heat production may be used as part of the greatly increased maintenance requirement and therefore may not appear as additional heat. It takes the place of some of the heat that the animal must otherwise produce to maintain its body temperature. At high temperatures, even in animals that are not growing or producing milk or eggs and that are therefore at the maintenance level of nutrition, the heat increment of feeding requires dissipation. Environmentally derived heat is added to the metabolic heat, which includes heat derived from activity, so that the total heat load requiring dissipation can be considerable.

Another disadvantage of hot regions is the high level of disease and parasite infestation. This is one factor that has led to unsatisfactory results in transferring such animals as cattle, sheep, and poultry from a

123

temperate to a hot climate. Growth rates, milk yields, egg production, and fertility all decline as a result of disease and lack of heat tolerance. Native breeds of animals are far better adapted to the environment and are more resistant to disease, but their levels of productivity are lower than those of selected animals raised in temperate climates.

Hot Regions

The hot regions of the world fall into two principal categories: the wet tropics and the deserts.

Tropics

Much of the earth's surface between 23° north and south of the equator is hot and humid and constitutes the tropics. These areas generally have two rainy seasons and two relatively dry seasons; air temperatures move between 22°C and 32°C, and the relative humidity is 50 percent during the day and approaches 100 percent at night. Although food is abundant and shelter is unnecessary for wild animals, the combination of uniformly warm environments and high humidities does not favor animal production. An additional disadvantage is the unchanging daylength, because coat changes, reproductive cycles, and metabolism are linked to photoperiodic seasonality. However, tropical zones, with their high rainfall and rich vegetation, do provide less direct solar heat load than the desert and support buffalo and beef cattle as productively used domestic animals (Moule, 1968). Indian cattle have been used extensively as meat-producing animals in Brazil; buffalo are indigenous to India, Burma, and Malaya, and there are many in China, where they are used for draft purposes and sometimes for milk.

Deserts

The deserts of the world are found in the latitudes from 15° to 32° north and south of the equator. They fall into three classes, cold, warm, and hot, all characterized by low rainfall and sparse vegetation. What vegetation does exist is scattered, and in the hot desert livestock are affected adversely by high daytime air temperatures and very high solar radiation levels, which can reach more than 1000 W/m^2. The arid regions occupy about 20 percent of the world's land surface, and the semiarid constitute a further 15 percent.

Although it is true that the primary characteristic associated with "desert" is relative lack of water, to consider the climate of the world's deserts only in terms of water shortage is to make an incomplete assessment. The survival of animals and plants in the desert depends on their ability to keep cool and to avoid desiccation and is influenced to a large degree by the 24-hourly fluctuation in temperature. This can be very marked, reaching 30°C or more in amplitude. This fluctuation is produced by clear skies with high intensities of solar radiation during the day and a high rate of reradiation from the earth's surface at night. The consequences are high air and surface temperatures during the day, and low air and surface temperatures that may approach freezing during the night. When the night temperatures fall below the dewpoint condensation occurs and water reaches the soil. An example of this effect is the growth of vegetation that occurs around telegraph posts in the desert; the growth is made possible by water condensing on the cooled post at night and running down to the ground.

Deserts, with their lack of water and plants, are clearly not compatible with considerable animal production, but many semi-desert areas in Africa, America, the middle east, Asia, and Australia are used for animal production. These areas merge with semiarid scrubland, which maintains numbers of ruminants. Sheep, in particular, exist in a very wide range of climates and they are important in hot, semiarid regions in China, northern Africa, and the middle east.

adult man's critical temperature is about 27°C. The change in thermal environment required for comfort and survival in the course of the pig's life is thus much greater than it is for man.

Adaptation of Domestic Animals to Heat

Adaptation to high temperatures involves physiological, behavioral, and morphological changes, primarily in patterns of heat dissipation through both the nonevaporative and the evaporative channels, but secondarily also in metabolism, including diminished levels of feed intake. Some of these modifications can be illustrated in different species. For example, as environmental temperature rises, feed consumption by Brahman cattle begins to decline at 32°–35°C and by Jerseys at 26°–29°C. Brahman cattle have a lower metabolic rate than European cattle and make more efficient use of ingested food. Their rates of weight gain under hot conditions exceed those of European cattle. These characteristics make the Brahman well adapted to existence in hot climates.

Different ranges of thermal adaptation during the course of growth can be seen by comparing the pig and man. The newborn pig is susceptible to cold; only as it grows does it become increasingly susceptible to heat, and its ambient temperature requirements change more than they do in the case of man. The newborn pig has a critical temperature of about 34°C, and the newborn baby one of about 35°C (Mount, 1966). At 34°C, without a wallow or other water to make up for its lack of sweating, the mature pig becomes distressed and may die in hyperthermia; at 35°C, although he is uncomfortable, adult man can survive indefinitely. The mature pig's critical temperature may fall to 0°C or even lower (Irving, 1964);

Adaptation to Heat

In a hot dry environment, the importance of water economy is paramount. Many animals are equipped with efficient mechanisms of sweating or panting that keep the body temperature within limits even in very hot environments. One of the consequences of evaporative cooling is the loss of water, which under extreme conditions can lead to dehydration, discussed below. Animals exhibit various types of adaptation by which dehydration is avoided. Some animals adopt a nocturnal habit, and so avoid the heat of the day by sheltering in their burrows. In the camel, the body temperature rises during the day and falls at night, which reduces heat dissipation. In both cases evaporative loss is lessened. Man in the desert has chosen to adopt loose clothing, which provides shelter from radiant heat during the day and protection against cold at night (Chapter 10). Some of the characteristic morphological adaptations in domestic animals are given in Table 9–1, and some metabolic features of desert ungulates in Table 9–2. These topics have been considered extensively by Macfarlane (1964; 1968a,b).

Pigs kept in warm environments develop longer limbs and larger ears than animals of the same breed kept in the cold. Subtropical cattle have dewlaps and long limbs. The dewlap has been considered to act as a heat dissipator by adding to the animal's surface area, but it has no greater concentration of sweat glands than other parts of the body. It is by increased sweating that any advantage accrues in the heat, because for sensible heat flow at high air temperatures an increased surface area leads to

Table 9–1   Main Morphological, Anatomical, and Functional adaptations
in Domestic Animals[a]

Environmental stress	Adaptive mechanisms	Animal (breed)
Solar radiation	Long limbs	Camel
	Short reflecting coat	Gazelle
High temperature	Hair shedding in summer	Ungulates
	Increased surface area in skin folds	Cattle (Brahman)
	Small body, long ears	Donkey
	Loose, coarse wool	Sheep (Awassi)
	Fine, dense wool	Sheep (Merino)
High humidity	Dark pigmentation, sparsely haired	Buffalo
Low temperature	Long hair intermixed with fine hair	Cattle (Scottish Highland)
	Minimum exposed extremities	Yak (Tibetan)
	Good grazing behavior	Musk ox (Arctic)
	Thick subcutaneous fat	Arctic species
	Abundant brown fat	Neonate of several mammals
	Thickset, heavy coat	Horse (Shire)
Seasonality in available feed	Ruminant stomach	Ungulates
	Adipose tissue reserves—hump(s)	Camel
	Adipose tissue reserves—fat tail	Sheep (Awassi, Kurdi, Masai, Karakul)
	Adipose tissue reserves—fat rump	Sheep (Somali, Sudan, black-head)
	Adipose tissue reserves—in rumen	Antelope

Deserts
  thorny vegetation
  water scarcity
	Thick skin, hard tissue around mouth	

	Thick mouth, lined with long papillae	
	Increased drinking capacity	Camel
	Hump (for pseudo water storage)	
	Conservation of metabolic water	
	Ability to survive dehydration	
High altitude	Increased O_2 carrying power in blood through increased concentration of red blood cells	
	Ability to transfer O_2 from capillary blood to tissue cells at a lower partial pressure	Llama, alpaca
	High efficiency in extracting nutrients from feeds	

[a] From Hafez (1968c). In *Adaptation of domestic animals,* Lea and Febiger, Philadelphia, p. 72.

greater heat transfer to the animal from the environment, rather than increased heat loss. Investigations on Red Sindhi bulls before and after surgical removal of the dewlap have shown no marked differences in response to heat, so the value of the dewlap for heat loss under conditions of thermal stress is questionable (McDowell, 1972).

Desert sheep also have long limbs, long ears, and long tails. Typically they also have local stores of fat, chiefly as either a fat tail or a fat rump (see Table 9–1). There are also local deposits of fat on the neck and dewlap in Masai and Blackhead sheep. The humps of the camel contain a fat store, varying with the food supply, and fat may constitute 30 percent of the body weight of cattle.

Under hot conditions, animals tend to become nocturnal in habit; this is the case in the tropics and subtropics. Animals seek shade from hot sun; if shade is not available they turn themselves to present the smallest bodily profile area to the sun. The pig seeks out shaded wet spots in hot weather and wallows in mud, which effectively compensates for the animal's inability to sweat. Reactions to thermal stress can be different in breeds of the same species. For example, European cattle do not use behavioral adjustments for temperature adaptation between 2°C and 21°C, whereas the corresponding range for Brahman cattle extends into the warmer levels of 10°–27°C (Hafez, 1968b).

Thermoregulation

Thermoregulatory control normally operates to keep a mammal's deep body temperature at a remarkably stable level, within limits, under a variety of conditions of environment and activity. If the body temperature is forced up by any means, including activity and feeding at high environmental temperatures, death occurs when a point between 42°C and 45°C is reached.

The animal's responses to heat serve to protect it from lethal hyperthermia unless conditions are extreme. These responses fall into several categories, which are discussed in detail elsewhere in this book: decreasing heat production (Chapter 2), increasing heat loss, including evaporative loss; decreasing thermal insulation (Chapters 2, 3, and 4); and behavioral reactions (Chapter 7). There is considerable evidence that thyroid activity

Table 9–2. Main Features of Desert Ungulates That Help Survival in Arid Regions[a]

Protection from heat, radiation, or cold	Short reflecting coat	Gazelle
	Light color	Eland
	Thicker coat in winter	Zebu cattle, Sudan and Somali sheep, donkey, camel
	Wool	
	loose, coarse	Awassi sheep
	fine, dense	Merino sheep
Evaporative cooling	Apocrine sweating	Camel, donkey
	Sweating and respiratory evaporation	Zebu, Merino
Metabolism	Lowered during dehydration	Camel
	Relatively low and low when heated	Merino, Zebu
Reserves	Fat stores	Camel, Zebu
	hump	Awassi, Kurdi, Masai, and Karakul sheep
	fat tail	
	fat rump	Somali, Sudan and blackhead sheep
	Water	
	alimentary reserve, mainly	Camel, cattle
	rumen extracellular volume	Sheep
Water and urea economy	Water	
	low renal flow normally	Camel
	low renal flow during dehydration	
	colon water reabsorption	Sheep
	Urea	Zebu
	renal reabsorption	Camel, sheep, Zebu
Behavior	Feed in the sun	Antelope, camel, Zebu, Merino
	Eat xerophytes, thorns, and salt plants	Antelope, goat, camel, donkey, sheep
	Feed without water	Camel, donkey, Zebu, Merino
	Active walkers between waterings	Antelope, camel, Zebu, blackhead Persian and Somali sheep, donkey, Merino

[a] The tabulation lists ungulate types in the approximate order of adaptation achieved to desert conditions. Where there are no observations, animals have not been included. From Macfarlane (1964).

is reduced in the heat and that both birds and mammals adapted to hot climates have reduced metabolic rates, accompanied by decreased activities of oxidative enzymes (Chaffee and Roberts, 1971). When cattle are exposed to moderate heat, the rate of heat production falls during the course of several days; the fall is associated partly with a fall in feed intake. At 32°C, the feed consumption of lactating Holstein cattle falls by 20%, and at 40°C it declines to zero and rumination decreases. High temperatures reduce daytime grazing and the animals spend much time in the shade (Yousef et al., 1968). Thermal insulation is decreased, particularly by vasodilatation and increased blood flow in the skin of the extremities and ears, which have relatively little hair cover

and a high surface area for their volume. These factors increase heat transfer between animal and environment. Vasodilatation under a heavy coat contributes little to heat exchange because the consequent decrease in internal insulation is only a small proportion of the total insulation.

The rectal temperature in cattle is normally in the region of 39°C; it is raised during feeding and activity and falls after the ingestion of large quantities of cold water. It is also affected by acclimatization; prolonged exposure to heat leads to smaller rises in rectal temperature, respiratory rate, and heart rate in response to heat stress. Figure 9–1 shows this effect on temperature in three calves exposed to 45°C for 5 hours on each of 21 successive days. Most of the acclima-

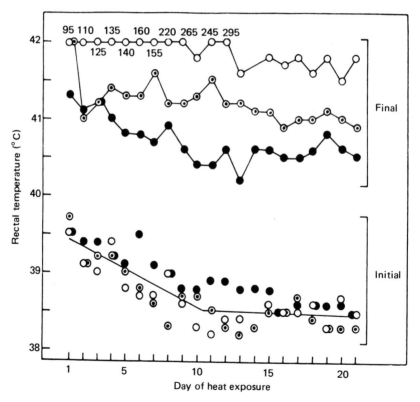

Fig. 9–1. Initial and final rectal temperatures of three calves exposed to 45°C dry bulb, 28°C wet bulb temperature for periods of up to 5 hours on each of 21 successive days. The figures on the top curve indicate the time in minutes taken by the least heat-tolerant calf to reach a rectal temperature of 42°C (Bianca, 1959, *J. Agric. Sci., Cam.,* **52:** 296).

tization occurs in the first 10 days, with a progressively falling initial rectal temperature before the heat exposure. The differences between the responses of the three animals indicate the range of heat tolerance to be expected within a population of calves. Such acclimatization is associated with decreased food intake, lower levels of thyroid activity and heat production, and thinning of the coat (Bianca, 1968).

Animal Coats

An animal's coat is of great importance not only in preventing excessive heat loss in the cold but also in preventing excessive heat gain under hot conditions. The three main types of coat are loose, tightly packed, and short smooth, and their efficiencies as insulators depend on the degrees to which they trap still air and how much radiation can penetrate. The sun's rays penetrate the loose coat of the Awassi sheep and produce a relatively high skin temperature, although the open nature of the coat allows much of the absorbed radiant energy to be lost by convection. The tightly packed coat of the Merino sheep reradiates in the long wavelengths when it is heated, and the short smooth coats of the goat and *Bos indicus* reflect solar radiation and allow convective loss (Fig. 9–2). With its thick highly insulating fleece, the Merino sheep reradiates some of the absorbed solar radiation as long-wave radiation to the surroundings from a wool surface that may reach 85°C. Some is lost by convection; the wool insulation maintains a temperature gradient of up to 43°C between the wool surface and the skin. In the equatorial camel, *Bos indicus,* and gazelles, the coat is short and smooth and much of the incident energy is reflected. This results in a skin temperature that is lower than otherwise expected, an effect that is increased by sweating.

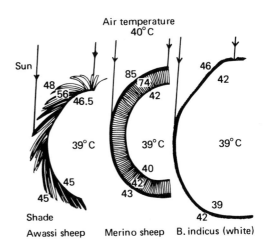

Fig. 9–2. Thermal behavior of the coats of Awassi sheep (loose, open fleece), Merino sheep (dense fleece) and Brahman cattle (short, shiny hair coat). The Awassi depends on convection for most of the heat loss, the Merino loses much of the incoming solar radiation by long-wave reradiation, and the Brahman reflects solar energy. Numbers without units are temperatures in °C (Macfarlane, 1968a).

In these three examples, the individual combinations of adaptations are different, involving dissipation of the solar radiant heat load by convection, reradiation, and reflection. The largest residual heat load that reaches the skin occurs in the Awassi sheep, with rather smaller loads in the Merino sheep and camel. These heat loads, together with the metabolic heat loads, must be dissipated by evaporation if thermoregulation is to be maintained (although changes in body temperature in the camel allow partial retention of the heat load during the day and its dissipation by nonevaporative means by night). The most effective desert animals are white, cream, or sandy in color, with a pigmented skin that probably offers protection against penetration by solar radiation. There is more reflection of solar radiation by lighter colored coats than by black, so that a light coat has a lower temperature in sunlight than a dark coat. About two-thirds of the incident heat, or more if there is a wind, is prevented by physical means from adding to the heat load of the organism.

Macfarlane (1964) has drawn up a heat balance for a Merino sheep of 1 m² surface area (and see Fig. 9–3):

Input	Watts	Output	Watts
Metabolic heat	45	Free convec-	70
Conduction from air	0	tion in still air	
Radiation from sun	280	Long-wave radiation	220
Radiation from sky	70	Total non-evaporative heat loss	290
Radiation from ground	60		
Total heat load	455		

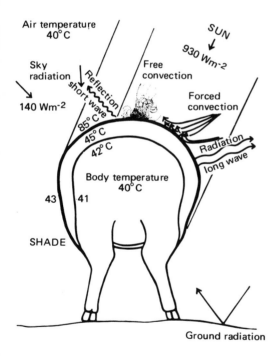

Fig. 9–3. Physical aspects of heat regulation by the fleece of a Merino sheep. Convection takes place both by the upward passage of heated air and by wind action. Radiation is to some extent reflected, but energy absorbed in the outer 1 cm of fleece induces temperatures of 85°–92°C in still air. This energy is lost by long-wave radiation to the sky (Macfarlane, 1968a).

In still air, therefore, there is a possible net heat gain of 165 W, much of which may be removed by wind convection. The relatively bare areas of face, legs, and tail may take up more heat, however. Fleece surface temperatures of 85°C or even more are reached in still air, and heat that is not lost by convection, long-wave radiation, and reflection passes through the fleece to the skin, which is at a temperature of about 42°C. The fleece is an excellent insulator because it is composed of nine parts of trapped air and one part of wool fiber. The surface characteristics of the fleece, together with its insulative value, allow the return of most of the incident heat to the environment. The net sensible heat gain must be dissipated through the evaporative channel.

Wind increases heat removal from the fleece. A fleece with a surface temperature of 90°C in still air has this reduced to 60°C within a few minutes by a wind of 5 m/second. As there is commonly a wind of this speed during the hot part of the day in the desert, wind is an important component of the environment in relation to an animal's tolerance of desert conditions. The cooling effect of wind is reduced by a rise in humidity, and a high vapor pressure in the atmosphere also decreases net long-wave radiation loss from the surface, so that such loss is lower in the humid tropics than in the desert.

When a Merino sheep is shorn, the albedo (ratio of the total luminous flux reflected to that received) increases from about 0.4 to 0.7, and the reflected sunlight increases to about 250 Wm⁻². In spite of this increased reflection, the total energy absorbed is two to three times that when there is a 5-cm fleece, in the case of a sheep in the open, although in shade shearing assists cooling by increasing convective loss (Macfarlane, 1968a). In sheep with loose fleeces exposed to intense solar radiation, the highest temperatures occur below the surface, where a zone of heated still air develops. In animals with hairy fleeces, and in the goat, the coat is reflecting, and surface temperatures rarely rise above 50°C. The hairy coat does not trap heat or water, so that evaporative heat loss is effective.

In cattle there is a 40 percent greater reflection of solar radiation from a white coat than from a black coat of the same length or texture. The long-wave emission is not affected by color, because with long waves all colors approach black body characteristics, with an emissivity close to unity. The black pigment found in the skin of tropical animals with short coats prevents the ultraviolet penetration that presents a survival hazard in the intense sunlight and clear atmospheres of the dry subtropics.

Evaporative Heat Loss

The primary partition of an animal's heat loss to the environment into evaporative and sensible components and the varying degrees to which different species can dissipate heat evaporatively by panting or sweating imply that the various components of the environment affect different animals to differing extents. This can be illustrated in the case of man, cattle, and pigs when the effects of a hot environment on body temperature in the three species are related to the dry bulb (DB) and wet bulb (WB) temperatures (Ingram, 1965a). The appropriate weightings of these two temperatures are as follows:

man: (DB × 0.15) + (WB × 0.85)
cattle: (DB × 0.35) + (WB × 0.65)
pigs: (DB × 0.65) + (WB × 0.35)

The high WB coefficient found for man reflects the significance of the ambient humidity in the considerable evaporative cooling process associated with the high density of sweat glands in the skin. The pig, which is unable to sweat effectively, has a correspondingly low WB coefficient, and cattle are intermediate between pig and man.

Under hot conditions, the pig makes up for its inability to sweat by wallowing in any

water or mud available, including urine and feces. The rate of evaporation from the skin surface then becomes comparable with the very high rates of sweating seen in man in the heat, and thermoregulation is very effectively maintained (Fig. 9–4). Under hot dry

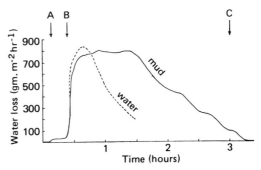

Fig. 9–4. Evaporative water loss from the skin of a pig measured by the ventilated capsule technique. At A, the capsule was placed on the skin. At B, mud (continuous line) or water (interrupted line) was smeared over the skin. At C, the capsule was removed (Ingram, 1965b).

conditions, however, the animal is at a great disadvantage because the rate of heat loss available to it through the respiratory evaporative channel is inadequate for thermoregulation.

Evaporative heat loss increases under hot conditions, both from the skin surface and from the upper respiratory tract, with differences between species in respect to the channel that is quantitatively the more significant. In man and cattle, for example, increased evaporative loss under hot conditions takes place primarily from the skin, whereas in the sheep and pig it is the respiratory evaporative loss that is more important. Sweating is associated with a cooler skin and a lower respiratory rate, whereas panting is associated with a warmer skin.

The relative importance of respiratory evaporation and sweating in relation to other factors involved in heat loss is indicated in Table 9–3. The table shows the complementary roles of respiratory and cutaneous water

Table 9–3. Ruminants Exposed to Heat and Sun during Summer in the Wet or Dry Tropics Show Various Combinations of Coat Protection, Cooling Mechanisms, and Water Conservation[a,b]

	Coat		Evaporative cooling		Water conservation		
	Reflec-tance	Insula-tion	Respira-tory	Sweat-ing	Renal	Fecal	Skin color
Merino sheep	+	+++	+++	+	++	++	White
Hair sheep	++	++	++	++	++	++	Dark
Goat	++	+	++	++	++	++	Dark
Bos taurus Shorthorn	++	+	++	++	+	+	White
Bos indicus Bibos banteng	+++	±	+	+++	+	++	Black
Buffalo	−	−	+	+++	+	+	Black
Camel							
subtropical	++	+	−	+++	+++	+++	Black
equatorial	+++	±	−	+++	+++	+++	

[a] From Macfarlane (1968b).

[b] (+++) Major effect, high efficiency; (++) moderate activity; (+) some effect; (±) very little action; (−) no action.

loss: as the one decreases, so the other increases in the list of species given. Rapid panting is characteristically shallow, with the result that air is moved to and fro over the turbinates, leading to evaporation from the mucosa and cooling of the blood flowing through the region. The higher the body weight, the lower the panting frequency; for example, in the adult Merino the rate rarely exceeds 350 per minute, whereas in the lamb the rate reaches 450 per minute (Macfarlane, 1968a). Normal lambs pant and sweat, but panting is the major route of heat loss in the hot zones of the world (Alexander, 1974).

In the sheep's upper respiratory tract the turbinate system is well developed, with the result that in the summer desert a sheep that has a facial skin temperature of 42°C has a surface temperature of 34°C over the turbinate bones because of dry air movement over the wet mucosa. Whereas in sheep only about one-eighth of evaporative cooling takes place through sweat gland activity, in cattle the roles of respiratory tract and sweat glands are reversed. At an air temperature of 38°C, Brahman cattle lose 12 percent of their evaporation from the respiratory tract compared with 24 percent in the Shorthorn,

and in the Brahman there is a much smaller increase in ventilation. Below 32°C, Brahman cattle vaporize less than European, an observation that is in keeping with their lower rates of heat production. Brahman cattle reach maximal vaporization rates at 35°C, whereas for European cattle the maximum is at 27°C. Respiratory cooling in cattle therefore provides only a small part of the evaporative heat loss, although cattle have well-developed turbinates. The partition of evaporative water loss between the respiratory tract and the sweat glands in adult sheep and cattle is given in Table 9–4. The water buffalo has only about one-sixth the number of sweat glands per unit area of skin as cattle and, like the pig, must rely on wallowing for wetting the skin under hot conditions.

Dehydration

The importance of evaporative cooling in thermoregulation in the heat draws attention to the availability of water and to the consequences of dehydration. The total body water of mammals living in hot climates usu-

Table 9–4. Partition of Evaporative Water Loss between the Respiratory Tract and the Sweat Glands in Adult Sheep and Cattle[a]

	Sheep	Cattle
Density of sweat glands (No./cm^2)	260–300	800–1500
Sweat gland volumes (mm^3)	0.001–0.008	0.006–0.015
Maximum sweat secretion rate (gm m^{-2} hr^{-1})	32	230
Maximum respiratory evaporation (gm m^{-2} hr^{-1})	95	41
Maximum evaporative cooling (kcal m^{-2} hr^{-1})	74	155
Respiratory rate per min (air temperature 40°C)	260	170

[a] From Macfarlane (1968a).

ally exceeds 70 percent of body weight; in temperate regions, where animals are fatter, the percentage water content is less than this. Cattle in the wet tropics have as much as 85 percent of body weight as water; equatorial sheep, 75 percent; and Merino sheep in the hottest part of Australia, 74 percent.

A discussion of dehydration in such large domestic animals as cattle and sheep is complicated by the large capacity of the rumen, which in a cow can hold 100 liters of water. In the ruminant the gut contents, which may form 20 percent of the body weight, are 85 percent water. In the study of the cow referred to by Bianca (1968), the animals were deprived of water for 2 days at 40°C. They lost 12 percent of body weight, 95 percent of which was water loss. The dehydration was associated with a decrease in the output of urine and feces, both of which reduced water loss. Although there was evidence of fluid loss from the blood for a given percentage loss of body weight, how-ever, the total solids in the serum increased by only half the value observed in man, probably because the large reservoir of water present in the rumen made an excessive demand on blood fluid unnecessary. During dehydration, the body temperature at which sweating began was slightly higher than in control animals. Table 9–5 gives some indication of relative losses of water through different channels in ungulates adapted to a dry existence.

Sheep, which are relatively tolerant of heat, can withstand a weight loss of up to 30 per cent under natural hot conditions when deprived of water for 5 days. Some of this water is probably derived from the rumen, but sheep are also capable of withstanding considerable reductions in plasma volume without failure of the circulatory system. Camels and donkeys also exhibit marked tolerance of dehydration, exemplified by their survival of a water loss of 27–32 percent of their body weight.

Table 9–5. Relative Loss of Water by Various Routes among Ungulates Adapted to Dry Country[a]

	Respiratory	Percutaneous	Renal	Fecal
Camelidae	±	+++	+	+
Equidae	±	++++	++	++
Bovidae	++	+++	+++	+++
Ovidae	++++	+	++	++

[a] Quantitative data are not standardized so that only relative amounts are shown, as in Table 9–3. Water elimination takes place in different proportions through the various routes. Camels and llamas do not increase respiratory water loss to any extent when heated, whereas Zebu cattle show some increase. European cattle have moderate respiratory cooling, whereas sheep evaporate most of the water for heat regulation from the nasal cavities. From Macfarlane (1964).

Goats use less water than sheep, and sheep use only about half as much as cattle (Macfarlane, 1968a). Some of the exchange characteristics for heat and water in sheep and cattle are given in Table 9–6. The figures for water turnover indicate a lower water requirement in *Bos indicus* than in *Bos taurus*, but both have considerably higher requirements than sheep. The water turnover can be defined as the amount of water passing through an animal in unit time, and it can be measured using a marker, such as tritiated water. Sheep and goats can live in temperate climates without drinking because their turnover rates for water are low. Cattle, however, with their higher turnover rate, must have water even under cool conditions. The half-time for turnover of water in the subtropics is 8 days for camels, 4 days for sheep, and 2.5 days for cattle. Equilibration of water throughout the cells and body fluids is slower in ruminants than in monogastric animals.

Cattle produce less concentrated urine than sheep, and their decreased power of water reabsorption in the colon and kidney is in keeping with their higher degree of dependence on ingested water and their greater daily excretion. Kidney structure is related to the animal's need for water. The kidney contains both long and short Loops of Henle, the proportion of the two types varying with the species. The more long Loops of Henle there are in the renal medulla, the greater is the potential reabsorption of water and the higher is the possible urine concentration. Cattle have mainly short loops and sheep have mainly long loops. The upper concentration limit reached in cattle urine is about 2.6 osmoles/liter, whereas in Merino sheep urine it is 3.5–3.8 osmoles/liter (Macfarlane, 1968b). These concentrations are reached during water deprivation; in normal life, concentrations over 1.5 osmoles/liter are rare. Cattle readily produce a diuresis after drinking, but sheep require a considerable water load (3 percent of body weight) for such an effect; camels can retain water without a diuresis. Camels have low initial glomerular filtration rates, of about 60 ml kg^{-1} min^{-1}, which fall to 15 ml kg^{-1} min^{-1} when water is restricted. In cattle and sheep, filtration rates are between 90 and 150 ml kg^{-1} min^{-1} and fall in dehydrated animals to one-third of this.

Merino sheep are intermediate between camels and cattle in their ability to survive water deprivation under hot conditions. During the first day at 40°C day temperature and 25°C night temperature, cattle lose 10

Table 9–6. Comparison of the Heat Input and Evaporative Cooling of Sheep and Cattle in Adaptation to Hot Environments[a]

	Hair sheep	Wool sheep	*Bos taurus*	*Bos indicus*
Surface temperature in sun (°C)	56	92	58	46
Reflectance of coat	++	+	+	+++
Long-wave emission	+	+++	++	+
Skin color	White	White	White	Black
Water turnover (ml $kg^{-0.82}$ per 24 hours)	180	220	530	400
Evaporative cooling sweating/respiratory ratio	0.2	0.12	4	6
Water reabsorption				
colon	+++	+++	+	++
kidney	+++	+++	+	++
Loops of Henle	Long	Long	Short	Short

[a] From Macfarlane (1968a).

Table 9–7. Relation of Body Fluids to Survival of Ruminants without Water in Desert Environments with Daily Maximum Temperatures of 40°C[a]

Phenomena	Camel	Merino sheep	Shorthorn cattle
Rate of weight loss (% per day)	2.0	4.5	7.0
Percentage of fluid lost from plasma	4.5	8.0	10.0
Days survival at maximum temperature = 40°C	12–15	6–8	3–4
Maximum urine concentration (osmoles per liter)	3.8	3.1	2.6
Maximum fecal dehydration (% water)	38	45	60
Maximum plasma sodium (mEq per liter)	202	185	170
Water loss as % of weight lost	85	74	66
Initial water replacement as % of weight lost	60	72	84

[a] From Macfarlane (1968b).

percent of body weight, sheep 8 percent, and camels 4 percent. The water content of the feces only falls to 60 percent in cattle after 3 days without water, whereas in sheep fecal water is 45 percent after 6 days and in camels about 40 percent after 5 days. The relation of body fluids to the survival without water of ruminants in desert environments is given in Table 9–7. The Merino sheep, *Bos indicus*, and *Bos taurus* are compared in Table 9–8 with respect to water balance and heat. Although *Bos indicus* needs less water than *Bos taurus*, it still requires twice as much water as the sheep and camel.

Animal Productivity

Reproduction

The following information is taken from Hafez (1968a), who gives an account of various investigations in this field.

Seasonal variations involve not only changes in temperature but also changes in daylength, so that it is difficult to dissociate the effects of these two variables on reproduction. It does appear, however, that high

Table 9–8. Comparison of Features of Tropical or Desert Types of *Bos indicus* with Shorthorn or Hereford *Bos taurus* Bred for Temperate Climates and with Merino Sheep[a]

Function in hot environments	Ovis aries (Merino)	Bos indicus (Brahman)	Bos taurus (Shorthorn)
Coat	Wool	Short, shiny	Longer
Behavior in sun	(Long-wave radiation)	(Reflecting)	(Heat absorbing)
Sweat glands	Small +	Large +++	Smaller ++
Respiratory cooling	Important ++	Slight +	Moderate ++
Foraging in the sun	Common	Common	Rare
Range of foodstuff eaten	Restricted	Wide	Restricted
Rumen yield of metabolites	+++	+++	++
Intestinal absorption			
of metabolites	+++	+++	++
of water	+++	++	+
Efficiency of conversion	+++	+++	++
Metabolic rate and water turnover	Low	Higher	Highest
Response to vasopressin	+++	++	+

[a] From Macfarlane (1968b).
[b] (+++) Major activity; (++) moderate; (+) minor.

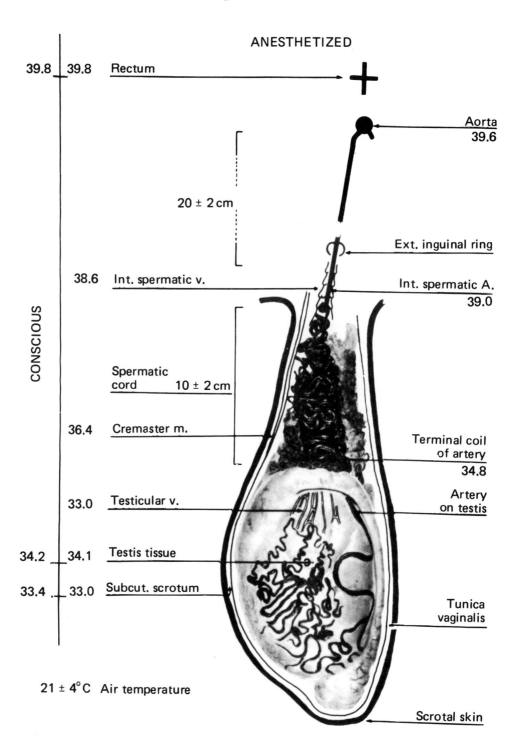

Fig. 9–5. Rectal, testicular, scrotal, and intravascular temperatures (°C) recorded in anesthetized rams. Corresponding temperatures in conscious rams are given to the left of the vertical line. Note the gradient temperatures (from Waites, G. M. H. and Moule, G., 1961, *J. Reprod. Fert.* **2:** 213).

temperatures do not affect the length of the estrous cycle in the sheep and pig, although in cattle the duration of estrus is shortened. Fertilization rate is reduced when sheep are exposed to 32°C before mating.

Testis Spermatogenesis in mammals is depressed at the deep body temperature. The thermoregulatory mechanisms in the scrotum, however, effectively produce a lower temperature in two ways (Fig. 9–5). First, the cremaster and dartos muscles hold the testes close to the body at low environmental temperatures, and allow the testes to drop when temperatures are higher. Second, countercurrent heat exchange (Chapter 3) takes place between the coiled artery and the veins, so that arterial blood reaching the testes is below body temperature.

Pregnancy High temperatures decrease fertility and litter size and increase abortion and fetal resorption. With ewes exposed to 42°C for 7 hours each day the embryos are damaged more when the animals are exposed throughout pregnancy than when they are exposed only in the latter half of pregnancy. Abortion has occurred in cows 4–6 months pregnant after a 27-hour exposure to 38°C. Pregnant cattle and sheep exposed to high temperatures produce small calves and lambs.

Lactation Above 27°C the milk yield in cattle declines markedly, but there are breed variations both in the levels of milk yield and in the temperature at which the decline begins (Figs. 9–6 and 9–7). The

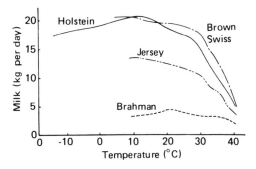

Fig. 9–7. Breed differences in the effect of environmental temperature on milk yield in cattle in a controlled temperature laboratory at relative humidity of 40–60% (Drawn by H. D. Johnson from data by Ragsdale et al., 1950, *Mo. Agric. Exp. Sta. Res. Bull.* Nos. 471 and 521, and taken from Hafez, 1968a).

associated decline in feed consumption is partly, but not entirely, the attributable cause of declining milk yield. The milk yields of a heat-intolerant cow and a heat-tolerant cow are similar at 18°C, but at 35°C the intolerant animal shows a decreased feed intake and decreased milk yield, whereas the tolerant animal's performance is unaffected. Milk yield per day decreases by approximately 1 kg for each 1°C rise in rectal temperature.

Figure 9–8 indicates the rates of water consumption for European and Brahman cattle, both lactating and nonlactating. Water consumption decreases at 32°C in lactating European cows, probably associated with declining milk production and feed consumption. Brahman cows continue to increase water consumption to a higher temperature, corresponding to the point at which their milk production and feed consumption decline. Nonlactating European cows show higher levels of water consumption than nonlactating Brahmans.

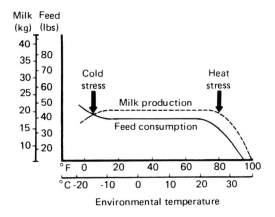

Fig. 9–6. Diagrammatic illustration of the effect of environmental temperature on milk production and feed consumption by cattle (By H. D. Johnson, from Hafez, 1968a).

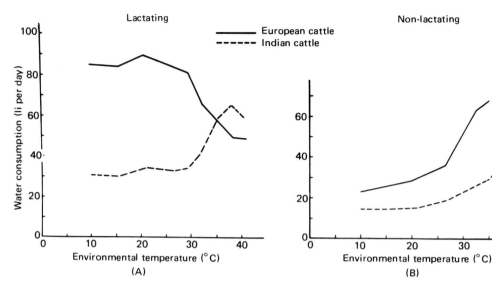

Fig. 9–8. Effect of environmental temperature on water consumption by (A) lactating and (B) nonlactating European (———) and Indian (– – –) cattle. (Data from Worstell and Brody, 1953, *Mo. Agric. Exp. Sta. Res. Bull.* No. 513; Johnson et al., 1963; *Mo. Agric. Exp. Sta. Res. Bull.* No. 846, and taken from Yousef et al., 1968).

Growth

Growth is depressed by high environmental temperatures, the effect varying with the breed. The consumption and digestibility of feed in the heat are both higher in Brahman than in European cattle, so that under hot conditions the rates of weight gain are higher in the former. In temperate regions, however, European cattle have higher growth rates than Brahman.

Selection for Hot Environments

For production in the tropics, animals should have a high efficiency of feed utilization, efficient heat loss mechanisms, and an ability to withstand some rise in body temperature and some dehydration, together with resistance to local diseases. The three approaches to this problem are (Yousef et al., 1968):

1. Selection within native breeds. This is feasible if the initial stock is productive.
2. Grading up by crossing with improved breeds. This has been used in South Africa and Egypt.
3. Development of new breeds. This is exemplified in the Santa Gertrudis breed of cattle, which is a Shorthorn–Brahman cross. This animal has the productive characteristics of the Shorthorn combined with the resistance to thermal stress shown by the Brahman. Another example is that of Russian crosses of native sheep with Merinos, which have led to productive animals that can survive and reproduce in conditions unsuitable for the Merino.

McDowell (1972), in his book on the improvement of livestock production in warm climates, considers that the genetic potential of many breeds of livestock that are native to hot countries is so limited that they cannot respond by increased productivity to improved environment and nutrition. He concludes that much wider use can be made of cross-breeding as a means of overcoming deficiencies in the native stock.

Desert Mammals

Large Mammals

The most famous of the desert mammals is the camel, and some aspects of its water economy have already been discussed. Stories of its capacity to survive for long periods without water abound, as do ideas about its capacity to store water. Schmidt-Nielsen (1964), who has studied this animal closely, has collected evidence from several sources, including the report of a journey lasting 21 days over 600 miles of waterless Sahara desert. The camel is a ruminant and its normal capacity for water is therefore large. However, Schmidt-Nielsen finds no evidence to support the idea that there are special "water sacs" in the stomach, nor is there evidence for a general higher tissue water content. He also points out that although the fat in the camel's "hump" represents a store corresponding to 40 liters of water that may be released during metabolism, this metabolism involves the use of oxygen that can only be gained by ventilating the lungs. This leads in turn to a loss of water from the respiratory tract when the animal breathes the very dry air of the desert. The camel's kidney, however, is capable of producing urine that is twice as concentrated as sea water. It is therefore possible for the animal to drink water that is more saline than other animals can tolerate and to eat plants with a high salt content. The feces are also very low in water content (about 40 percent; see Table 9–7) when water intake is low.

Schmidt-Nielsen has made observations on camels deprived of water and has found

them exceptionally able to withstand dehydration of up to 25 percent of body weight. Moreover, in the desert winter it takes 17 days for a camel to lose 16 percent of body weight, and even in summer 7 days are required to lose 25 percent. As soon as water is available, however, the animals can drink, without raising the head, almost exactly the amount of water they have lost, but no more. Of the water lost during dehydration about half comes from the gut. The contribution of the plasma is relatively small. Blood volume is reduced by only about 20 percent during dehydration, which means that compared with other species, such as man, the load placed on the circulatory system is not great.

One other adaptation exhibited by the camel that helps it to reduce water loss is its ability to allow fluctuations in its body temperature. Even when water is freely available, the 24-hour variation in body temperature is 2°–3°. Under conditions of dehydration, however, the temperature not only rises to a higher level during the day but also falls to a lower value at night. This increased fluctuation is associated with an increase in body temperature at which sweating begins and with a decrease in the threshold temperature for increased metabolism. The net result is that the camel can store much of the heat load it receives during the hot desert day and lose it by convection and radiation during the cool desert night (Schmidt-Nielsen, 1964). The daytime hyperthermia has the effect of sparing water that must otherwise be used for evaporative cooling. It may be regarded as an adaptation to high temperatures that takes place particularly when dehydration threatens. This adaptation is of particular value in larger animals, which have a larger heat capacity per unit surface area and consequently a higher ratio of heat storage potential to heat exchange with the environment than do smaller animals. It is seen, for example in the donkey which is another animal frequently used as a beast of burden under desert conditions. To some extent its body temperature also fluctuates under conditions of dehydration, although the daily variations are not as great as those of the camel. It can also produce a urine more concentrated than can man. Tolerance to dehydration is similar to that observed in the camel (over 25 percent of body weight) and, like the camel, it does not undergo the relatively large reduction in plasma volume seen in man.

Taylor (1972) has shown that in Thompson's and Grant's gazelles body temperature increases during dehydration. The threshold temperature for panting is also increased, particularly in Grant's gazelle, which extends its range into the hot arid regions of east Africa. This change in threshold can be demonstrated quite dramatically if the animals are exposed to 40°C. Normally hydrated animals pant; dehydrated ones do not but simply allow the body temperature to rise. Taylor has also shown that Grant's gazelle can thrive without water in places that have had no rain for 2 years. He found that although the plants available to the animal have a water content of only 1 percent during the day, they gain moisture by condensation from the air at night and their water content rises to as much as 30 percent. By grazing at night, therefore, the gazelle is virtually able to drink water out of the air. In a corresponding situation, Louw (1972) has described the dependence on fog water of certain water-storing beetles and lizards in the Namib desert on the southwestern coast of Africa. The fog, produced by a cold ocean current, also sustains succulent plants that support other animals which are well adapted to desert life but which do not store water, such as the ostrich and Namib gerbil.

Adaptations to desert conditions by two kangaroos, the red and the euro, have been described by Dawson (1972). Both animals live in the arid interior of Australia, but whereas the red kangaroo lives on the open plain, the euro lives in rocky hill country and uses caves as refuges from heat. Both animals have the low resting metabolic rates characteristic of marsupials. Their body temperatures at thermal neutrality are approximately 35.5°C, clearly lower than the level usually found in eutherian mammals. The red kangaroo is exposed to solar radiation, and its fur is not only nearly twice as reflective as that of the euro but is also more resistant to penetration by solar radiation. Another difference between the two animals is that the panting rate in the red kangaroo, at environmental temperatures of 35°–45°C, is much below that of the euro, although evaporative loss is higher in the red than in the euro. This apparent contradiction may be explained by a greater tidal volume in the red than in the euro, giving the red an equivalent evaporative loss for a lower respiratory frequency. Licking or wiping of saliva on to the forelimbs occurs in both animals during heat stress; it is more noticeable in the red kangaroo and this may produce this animal's higher water loss.

Rodents

The desert rodents lack sweat glands and avoid heat exposure; the small animal cannot afford to use water for thermoregulation because of its large surface area relative to its mass. Calculation of the necessary evaporative rate as a percentage of body weight shows that this is increasingly prohibitive as the animal becomes smaller (Fig. 9-9). Most burrows are at a depth of 0.5–1.0 m, where there is little temperature fluctuation: at a 0.5-m depth the daily fluctuation is about 1°C and at a 1-m depth it is zero. At the surface, however, the fluctuation may be of the order of 50°C, with the surface temperature rising as high as 75°C. The maximum temperatures in the burrows at the height of the summer are in the region of 29°–31°C.

Most desert rodents are nocturnal in habit and in this way avoid the daytime heat

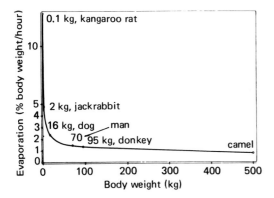

Fig. 9–9. Relation between body size and the evaporation estimated to be necessary for the maintenance of a constant body temperature in a hot desert climate (from Schmidt-Nielsen, 1954).

load. Those which are not primarily nocturnal adopt an intermittent type of activity pattern. The antelope ground squirrel, for example, spends a period above ground while its body temperature rises and then descends into its burrow and lies in close contact with the ground while its body temperature falls. If the animal is exposed continuously to 40°C it succumbs within a few hours.

The tolerance of desert rodents to hyperthermia is not exceptional; if the body temperature does approach the lethal limit of 42°–43°C, some desert rodents salivate excessively, spreading saliva over the body so that evaporative cooling can take place. This is an emergency measure however, for repetition must lead rapidly to fatal dehydration. Desert rodents may be divided broadly into two groups: those which conserve water, and those which live on food with a high water content. The water conservers include the jerboa, gerbil, and kangaroo rat. They use water produced by metabolism and take dry food with no added water; even when water is present the animal seldom drinks it. Water loss is diminished by reducing respiratory evaporative loss through countercurrent heat exchange in the upper respiratory tract (the kangaroo rat expires air at 24°C, so that water condenses on the mucosa during expiration), by producing a very concentrated

urine, and by excreting a small amount of very dry feces. In addition, the kangaroo rat practices coprophagy (eating its own feces), as do many other rodents, but in this instance the saving of water is involved. The only source of water to these animals is the metabolic water derived from the food, and Schmidt-Nielsen (1964) has shown how this is sufficient to keep the animal in water balance.

The other group of animals, which live on water-containing food, includes the pack rat, sand rat, and grasshopper mouse. The pack rat drinks no water but cannot withstand dehydration. This animal depends for food on cactus plants, which have a high water content, and its only metabolic adaptation appears to be the ability to utilize food that is toxic to the white rat. The pack rat's kidney, however, is less efficient at concentrating urine than that of the white rat (Schmidt-Nielsen, 1964).

Some desert rodents estivate; that is, they become dormant during the hottest and driest part of the summer. The body temperature usually falls to within 1°C of the ambient temperature, with a decreased metabolism and a consequent sparing of evaporative loss. Hibernation is another case of dormancy serving energy conservation, but in this case in the cold; many estivators also hibernate.

Birds

Whereas the domesticated mammals have deep body temperatures ranging from 36°C to 39°C, such temperatures in domestic birds range from 41.2°C to 42.2°C (Siegel, 1968). Birds native to hot environments have body temperatures not significantly different from those of temperate-zone birds; some, such as the ostrich, can maintain a near-normal body temperature of 39.7°C for several hours at an ambient temperature of

51°C (Chaffee and Roberts, 1971). The upper lethal body temperatures are similar for both desert and nondesert birds. For example, the chicken, during the first week of life, has a critical temperature of 34°C; this falls to 32°C when the bird is 5 weeks old and to 18°C when it is adult. The upper lethal body temperature is 47°C throughout life. However, unless food intake is controlled, the demonstration of the critical temperature is difficult (Richards, 1974).

Under hot conditions, birds lose heat by respiratory evaporation; there are no sweat glands. The air passages to the lungs communicate with the air sacs and so are open at both ends. The sacs allow areas of moist surface for evaporative cooling but do not take part in gaseous exchange. They also appear to function as air reservoirs during ventilation and as surfaces for limited CO_2 diffusion to the air (King and Farner, 1964). Panting occurs, with increased respiratory frequency and decreased tidal volume; open-mouthed panting begins when body temperature exceeds a value between 41°C and 44°C. Although tidal volume is decreased, respiratory alkalosis develops. The maximum respiratory frequency is 140–170 per minute in the chicken at a body temperature of 44°C; if body temperature rises further, respiration rate declines and tidal volume increases. The ostrich behaves more like a dog, changing abruptly from a low breathing rate to rapid panting. Panting may be controlled by a center in the midbrain. The influence of the hypothalamus is to facilitate panting, but it appears not to be essential for this function, because total destruction of the hypothalamus has not been shown to abolish panting in severe hyperthermia (Richards, 1974).

Some birds augment panting by rapid fluttering of the gular area, produced by flexing of the hyoid apparatus. The rate of gular flutter increases in some cases with the heat load; gular flutter increases evaporative heat transfer and convective loss by forced convection. Birds that are acclimatized to high temperatures have lower maximum respiratory frequencies, reduced hematocrit and plasma volume, and increased water intake. Several species of birds, not necessarily native to the desert, can dissipate all their metabolic heat by evaporative cooling at high environmental temperatures. Birds native to hot environments tend to have reduced resting metabolic rates. Under very hot conditions, in the middle of the day in north American deserts, birds retreat to shaded areas of rock crevices; soaring birds climb to great heights where the air temperature is lower and secondary radiation less marked (Dawson and Hudson, 1970).

The survival of birds in the desert appears to depend mainly on their capacity to tolerate rises in body temperature to about 4°C above the normal level and on behavioral adaptation, because they do not have special mechanisms for dealing with heat and dryness (Dawson and Schmidt-Nielsen, 1964).

Birds secrete uric acid instead of the urea of the mammal; uric acid is highly insoluble, and water is reabsorbed in the cloaca, the uric acid being lost as a paste with very little water. The production of uric acid rather than urea also means that birds produce about 20 percent more water from the metabolism of protein than do mammals. This does not mean that birds do not need to increase their water intake at high environmental temperatures, however, because the quantities involved in evaporative heat loss are very considerable. One economy is achieved by allowing a passive rise in body temperature so that the amount of water lost does not increase progressively at high ambient temperatures, as it does in mammals. The amount of heat that can be stored in this way is obviously limited in small birds. If deprived of water, however, the ostrich develops a greater hyperthermia when exposed to heat than do similar birds when they are drinking (Chaffee and Roberts, 1971).

In addition to the kidney, birds have a nasal gland that secretes a concentrated solution of sodium chloride and that is particularly well developed in marine birds.

Birds from the arid zones also seem to be able to tolerate salt in their drinking water, but there is no evidence to suggest that this is allowed by the activity of the salt gland, which is poorly developed in most terrestrial birds. In desert birds it appears that the kidney is particularly well equipped to deal with salt loading of the body.

With regard to bird productivity in the heat, thermal stress has an adverse effect on both egg weight and shell quality. Above 32°C, shell thickness decreases. The temperature of incubation influences the size of the blastoderm; development is retarded and somite formation is inhibited at temperatures below 35°C (Hafez, 1968a).

Poikilotherms

The dependence of the poikilotherm on the environment for its levels of body temperature and metabolic activity implies that the hot humid climate is most suited to it. This is borne out by the diversity and size of poikilotherms in such climates. The absence of internal autonomic control, however, does not prevent the use of behavior in controlling body temperature by varying exposure to different environments. Under hot dry conditions, desiccation is the chief danger to the poikilotherm. Various adaptations are seen in these species under hot conditions (Clarke, 1967; McWhinnie, 1967; Fry, 1967).

Reptiles

Although reptiles have no sweat glands, water loss through the skin may nevertheless be appreciable and respiratory activity may actually be increased under very warm conditions. Under less severe conditions, however, the high water content of the food, and

the elimination of uric acid yielding more water than when urea is excreted, enable the animals to maintain water balance.

The oxygen consumption of the reptile is lower than that of the desert rodent. The amount of water evaporated per unit of oxygen consumed is higher in the reptile than in the desert rodent, even though the expired air of the reptile is not saturated at so high a temperature as in the mammal. This difference favors diminished water loss in the reptile. The desert iguana, resting at 37°C and therefore with a body temperature similar to the mammal's, nevertheless has a metabolic rate only about one-seventh that of the desert rodent. One consequence of this is that the reptile produces much less metabolic water. The absolute rate of water loss from the reptile is less than that from the homeotherm at the same temperature.

Reptiles adopt several different modes of thermoregulation (Templeton, 1970). Many reptiles can maintain their body temperatures within controlled limits independently of environmental temperature. This is achieved by the behavioral use of sun and shade. Acclimation to temperature in most desert reptiles is not as important as behavioral control.

Some aquatic reptiles, including snakes and turtles, never leave the water, with the exception of female turtles depositing eggs. Their body temperatures therefore correspond with that of sea water.

The semiaquatic reptiles, notably the crocodile, leave the water to bask. The Nile crocodile basks in the hour before dawn, before air temperature rises above water temperature, and then retires to shade or to partial submersion. It reemerges to bask in the afternoon until just before sunset, when it returns to the water for the night.

Terrestrial reptiles may burrow or be active at night, and they may be thigmothermic or heliothermic. The thigmotherms do not bask, but they thermoregulate by heat exchange with the air or by contact with the ground. Heliotherms gain heat primarily from solar radiation. An extensively studied animal of this type is the desert lizard. Activity temperatures are reached by basking, and then during its activities the animal moves between sun and shade, so keeping body temperature relatively steady. As the day becomes warmer, less time is spent in the sun, until by midday all activity is in the shade. When conditions become warmer, the animal may partially bury itself in sand, so reaching cooler sand, and when too hot the lizard retreats underground. The desert iguana, before retreating underground, sometimes climbs bushes where the air is somewhat cooler than nearer the ground.

The critical maximum temperature is the body temperature at which a reptile, exposed to high temperatures, loses the capacity for coordinated movement. It dies as its temperature rises further, although it can survive the critical maximum temperature without permanent damage if removed from the exposure. The critical maximum temperature is therefore more important than the lethal temperature from the ecological standpoint. It is correlated with the habitat; among turtles it has been found to be lowest (41°C) in aquatic species, and highest (43.3°C) in terrestrial species. In general, lizards can withstand higher temperatures than snakes, and diurnal species can withstand higher temperatures than nocturnal forms. The critical maximum temperatures for lizards and snakes from the same area have been given as 45°–47°C and 42°C, respectively (Cloudsley-Thompson, 1971).

Amphibia

The skin of amphibia is permeable to water, and consequently these animals cannot be expected to present a high degree of resistance to dehydration. Their ability to exist in hot climates depends chiefly on the selection of a moist habitat.

Amphibia tend to be more cryophilic than reptiles; a temperature of 28°C kills some salamanders and frogs, although others can tolerate temperatures as high as 42.5°C. Two varieties of *Bufo boreas* that live in arid areas of California and Nevada show little acclimation, and the need for a moist environment makes the desert hostile to the amphibian.

Invertebrates

Soft-bodied animals, such as worms, which have a skin that is permeable to water, have little resistance to dehydration. The presence of a cuticle or shell may change the picture, for the snail can withdraw into the microclimate of its shell, which is sealed by the operculum, and under these conditions it loses very little water. Schmidt-Nielsen et al. (1972) have shown that snails living in the desert and feeding off the green growth that occurs in the winter may in fact be able to exist for 4 years without water at the very low rates of loss that occur while they are dormant.

Other invertebrates, such as woodlice and centipedes, may avoid problems of dehydration by the selection of suitable microclimates even under arid conditions. Once in a hot dry atmosphere, however, they rapidly succumb. The desert woodlouse digs holes of 5-mm diameter vertically downwards for tens of centimeters, with two animals often working together (Cloudsley-Thompson, 1970). Insects and arachnids have a wax layer that prevents loss of water by transpiration, and they can also absorb water from unsaturated air.

The most important behavioral adaptation of invertebrates, particularly annelids and arthropods, to the hot dry environment is burrowing. Some desert snails estivate in cracks in the ground or in fissures in rocks; during estivation the mouth of the shell is closed by a thick diaphragm that reduces evaporative loss. These behavioral reactions take the animals to favorable microclimates that are markedly different from the prevailing meteorological conditions. High lethal temperatures are characteristic of invertebrates that live in hot deserts; the scorpion, for example, has a lethal temperature of 47°C. In the case of desert beetles and scorpions, heat death appears to be caused primarily by the accumulation of acid waste products of metabolism. Diapause, a dormant resting phase, is widespread among desert arthropods; it is primarily an adaptation to drought rather than to high temperature (Cloudsley-Thompson, 1970).

CHAPTER 10

Man in Hot Environments

There are broadly two situations in which a man is exposed to hot conditions. In the first, the individual is accustomed to living in a hot environment; he is in equilibrium with it and adapted to it. He may live in the desert or in a tropical country, or he may live in a temperate climate and yet spend a part of each day at high temperatures, as in the case of a foundry worker. In each of these cases he is routinely exposed to heat. The second situation is when the temperature rises from the equable, cool level associated with his usual surroundings, and to which he is accustomed, to a height that imposes severe demands on his thermoregulatory mechanisms to the degree that adaptation is necessary. The adaptation includes initial acute responses, and, if exposure to heat continues, these are followed by more persistent, chronic changes that constitute acclimatization to the changed conditions. This second situation illustrates the effects of high temperatures better than does the first, equilibrium situation, because it involves change and therefore contrasts physiological responses occurring before, during, and after acclimatization. The responses of man to a hot environment are therefore approached in terms of adaptation to a rise in environmental temperature.

Acclimatization to Heat

It is a matter of common observation that when the weather suddenly becomes hot the individual may be overtaken by lassitude and by a relative inability to perform effectively tasks that are carried out at a high level of efficiency under cooler conditions. Clothing is discarded, sweating is noticeable, and the individual becomes irritable; physical work previously undertaken without effort now becomes a burden and may be accompanied by nausea and dizziness. After a few days, however, discomfort decreases as acclimatization, with both psychological and physiological adjustments, takes place.

The exposure of man to a hot environment implies exposure to a degree of heat stress. As the environmental temperature rises above the critical temperature (Chapter 3), successive degrees of heat stress move toward the limit that can be tolerated. The limit is perhaps most appropriately indicated by the inability to maintain a normal deep body temperature as the environment becomes hotter.

Bass (1963) has discussed acclimatization to heat in a man undertaking physical work. The effects produced by heat during work are much more pronounced than those in the sedentary individual. Physical work imposes an additional metabolic heat load. It therefore enhances the rise in body temperature and rate of sweating, producing a correspondingly greater initial displacement of the thermoregulatory equilibrium and larger adaptive responses. Bass describes an unacclimatized individual asked to walk at 3½ miles per hour for 1 hour at 49°C. The subject first experiences severe discomfort, then dizziness, nausea, and even collapse, accompanied by high deep body and skin temperatures, very rapid pulse, and an inadequate secretion of concentrated sweat. If the walk is repeated every day, limited as necessary to what is within the capability of the individual, dramatic improvement in the performance of the task takes place within a few days. Subjective discomfort lessens, body temperature and heart rate fall, and sweat becomes greater in volume and less concentrated; this is the classical picture of acclimatization to heat (Fig. 10–1). Acclimatization to heat begins with the first exposure, and then progresses rapidly. It can be induced by short daily bouts of work in hot conditions.

Acclimatization is more rapid in subjects in good physical condition, whose maximal work load can be reached quickly by daily increases. It is well developed in 4–7 days; even without further exposure, it may be retained for about 2 weeks before it is progressively lost, although sometimes the loss is much more rapid. The length of daily exposure required to bring about acclima-

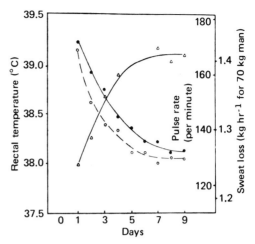

Fig. 10–1. Typical average rectal temperatures (●), pulse rates (○), and sweat losses (△) of a group of men during the development of acclimatization to heat. On day 0, the men worked 100 minutes at an energy expenditure of 350 W in a cool climate. The exposure was repeated on days 1–9 but in a hot climate with dry and wet bulb temperatures of 48.9°C and 26.7°C (Leithead and Lind, 1964).

tization has been the subject of investigation: 100 minutes in a single exposure is recommended as the most economical. There is no improvement in acclimatization with two such exposures a day (Leithead and Lind, 1964).

Acclimatization is often said to be specific for the conditions of exposure, both for the particular energy expenditure and for the particular environment. Under some conditions, acclimatization to one level of energy expenditure and one hot environment does not provide physiological adaptation either for a higher level of expenditure or for a hotter environment. However, acclimatization to work in a hot environment does occur in subjects whose body temperatures are raised passively by exposure to heat, using the technique of controlled hyperthermia, where work is not being undertaken. How much acclimatization is induced depends both on the duration of hyperthermia and on the elevation of body temperature (Fox, 1974).

Sweating

Exposure to heat results in an increased demand on the thermoregulatory system, and physical work under hot conditions increases the demand further. Evaporative heat loss provides the only effective channel for dissipating heat to the surroundings when the temperature of the surroundings is above that of the body. Under these conditions, nonevaporative heat transfer is an added heat load on the individual instead of a channel for heat dissipation.

In a cool environment, evaporative heat loss accounts for about 25 percent of the heat produced by the resting metabolism in man. As the environmental temperature rises, an increasing proportion of heat is lost by evaporation until, under hot conditions, this mode accounts for the total heat loss. As a result of his highly developed sweating function, man can withstand very high temperatures in a dry atmosphere (see reference to Blagden in Chapter 1).

A maximum sweating rate, up to 2 or even 3 kg hr^{-1}, can be achieved by individuals after full acclimatization, but only for short periods of time. Men working in the desert can lose 10–12 kg per day, and although urine output is reduced very rapidly it is obvious that extra water must be taken in if dehydration is to be avoided. That the quantity of sweat to be evaporated per hour for a constant body temperature to be maintained by a man under desert conditions at 40°C amounts to about 1.5 percent of the body weight indicates the magnitude of the problem.

In the unacclimatized man, in whom the sweat is concentrated and the loss of both water and salt leads to little osmotic imbalance, thirst does not always keep water intake up to the rate of loss. The heat-acclimatized man, however, produces a dilute sweat, loses relatively more water than salt, and is much more thirsty for a given water deficit and more nearly maintains his water

balance by voluntary drinking. When sweating at very high rates, man simply cannot drink water fast enough to keep in balance and efforts to do so may lead to vomiting.

A full explanation for this apparent shortcoming has not yet been found, but it is known that thirst is controlled by several factors. In the dog, water passing over the tongue partly offsets the apparent desire to drink, even when the water does not reach the stomach, but dryness of the mouth caused by ligation of the salivary ducts increases only the frequency of drinking and not the quantity drunk. Loading an animal with fluid via a gastric cannula influences the amount of water taken by mouth, depending on the salt concentration of the fluid; hypotonic liquids decrease water intake and hypertonic fluids increase intake. The degree of cellular hydration is another important factor.

Adolph (1947) has studied man subjected to a dehydration of 10 percent of body weight in the desert and has found that in spite of the severe thirst and mental derangement accompanying the maximum water deficit, recovery is complete within an hour of drinking. The signs of thirst are very strong when as little as 2 percent of body weight has been lost but do not get progressively worse as dehydration proceeds. After 4 percent weight loss the mouth is very dry, and at 8 percent the tongue is swollen and speech is difficult. Observations made on men who have been lost in the desert suggest that after a 12 percent loss of body weight recovery is possible only with some assistance, and it may be necessary to give water by injection or *per rectum*.

In a comparison between man and dog in the desert, Dill et al. (1933) have found that, in contrast to man, the dog drinks, at the first opportunity, almost the exact amount of water it has lost during a day in the desert. A second difference is that a differential loss of water from the plasma does not occur in the dog. The difference has been believed related to the fact that man loses large amounts of salt in the sweat and the dog does not. However, the differences persist even when a salt deficit in man is prevented by the provision of extra salt.

After exposure to extreme heat, dehydration in the dog follows a pattern similar to that in man. At a water loss of 14 percent of body weight there is an explosive rise in temperature that is lethal if dehydration is continued. By contrast, however, the dog can withstand as much as 17 percent dehydration in a cool environment. The reduced capacity to withstand dehydration in a hot climate is related to the reduced blood volume, which is no longer capable of transferring heat to the surface. The dog that is continuously exposed to a high temperature dies from circulatory failure, therefore, rather than from dehydration. The cat can withstand a slightly greater degree of dehydration than the dog, and the kidney can concentrate the urine to a greater extent, so that the animal is better able to withstand hot dry conditions.

According to dehydration studies in man, there appears to be very little tendency for sweat rate to diminish. A comparison of a group of men receiving water *ad libitum* and a similar group without water in the desert has shown that although the men without water use about 10 percent less water for cooling they become more dehydrated than the other group. The balance of the difference may possibly be accounted for by some economy of effort on the part of the dehydrated men. As Schmidt-Nielsen (1964) has pointed out, the idea that man may train himself to use less water during journeys in the desert is attractive but is based on wishful thinking rather than on sound physiological knowledge.

An important consequence of dehydration is that relatively more of the water lost as sweat is derived from the plasma than from other body fluids (Adolph, 1947; Robinson, 1949). A reduction of 3 percent in body weight through sweating is associated with a fall of 6.5 percent in plasma volume,

with a consequent increase in haematocrit and viscosity. The reason for this differential loss of water is not known. It is certainly not likely to be related to a rate-limiting factor in the exchange of water between tissues and blood, which is very rapid. Water must, in any event, be gained by the blood from the tissues almost as fast as it is lost, because in a single day the water loss can be greater than the total blood volume. Whatever the underlying cause, the consequent increased viscosity of the blood leads to increased work by the heart to maintain the circulation. Pulse rate increases and stroke volume decreases; the cardiac output remains about the same. This increased load on the heart occurs at a time when there is a large skin blood flow associated with heat-induced peripheral vasodilatation.

Although the amount of water lost as sweat decreases very little when man becomes dehydrated, body temperature nevertheless tends to rise. It is possible that this increase in temperature is related to a failing capacity of the blood to transport heat to the surface of the body, but it may represent a controlled rise in temperature similar to that which occurs during work. Such an increase in body temperature would be an advantage with respect to heat loss because the flow of sensible heat from the body is proportional to the temperature difference between the body and the surroundings. How far the rise in body temperature is a true adaptation to a hot environment and how far it is simply a fortuitous advantage has yet to be determined.

One obvious tendency that leads to economy in water is the reduction of urine flow by the excretion of a concentrated fluid. The extent to which this is possible, however, depends on the type of kidney; birds, for example, are able to produce a urine with an extremely low water content because water is reabsorbed in the cloaca. In man in a hot climate, urine volume is reduced to about half the usual quantity, even when water is freely available. If he is doing hard work, there is a further reduction, but the amount does not fall below about 500 ml/ day unless dehydration is very severe. The extent to which urine flow can be reduced depends on the ability of the kidney to concentrate the urine. In man, the ability to produce a concentrated urine is rather limited and is, for example, only about half that of the dog. Because sweat production, and therefore salt loss, is high in a hot climate, however, some salt is lost through the sweat glands. Under these conditions a slightly saline drinking water is an advantage in the maintenance of salt balance. The important factor, however, is the balance between the concentration of salt in the drinking water and the elimination of salt in the sweat. The drinking of concentrated urine is completely useless because the solutes are returned to the body and must be excreted again in just the same amount of water.

In preparation for a journey under desert conditions, perhaps the most important measure that a man can take is to dress in clothes that reduce the radiant heat load, and so reduce the quantity of heat that must be lost by evaporation. In comparison with the unclothed state, light clothes with long trousers and a long-sleeved shirt reduce radiant heat load by half and water loss by two thirds (Schmidt-Nielsen, 1964). Drinking as much water as possible before starting out on a journey in the desert is likely to lead to a diuresis unless the amount of antidiuretic hormone in the plasma is high. If conditions are already hot and sweat rate is high, however, some additional water can be drunk without affecting urine flow.

Sweat is more than 99 percent water, with variable amounts of sodium chloride as the principal constituent. The variations are related to the rate of sweating: in an unacclimatized man, as the rate increases, the concentration also increases, and the two quantities subside together. After frequent exposure to heat, however, although the rate of sweating increases, the chloride concentration decreases. In the summer, the concentration is lower and the sweating rate is higher; in the winter the reverse is true (Kuno, 1956; Ohara, 1972). In a hot environment, the chloride concentration falls in the urine as well as in the sweat and is therefore part of a more general salt-conserving adaptation in the heat. In individuals with a high level of chloride in the sweat, the decrease on adaptation to heat is slight, whereas in individuals with a low initial level the decrease occurs early. Folk (1966) quotes a chloride content of between 0.2 and 0.3 percent, with a few individuals at 0.1 or 0.6 percent. The actual salt loss in a hot environment may be as high as 15–20 gm per day and even higher under extreme conditions.

The maximum sweating rate occurring at rest was investigated by Kerslake and Brebner (1970). They heated subjects in a water bath until the mouth temperature was 38°C and then measured the sweat loss by weighing. Sweat rate was independent of mouth temperature provided this exceeded 38°C, but it varied with skin temperature, increasing by about 11 percent per °C rise (giving a Q_{10} of about 3). The maximum sweat rates were about 40 gm/minute for each of two subjects weighing 69 and 76 kg; the maximum rates were lower in the afternoon than in the morning.

Hey and Katz (1969) found active sweating in babies 0–10 days old, born within 3 weeks of the full term of the gestation period, when the environmental temperature exceeded 34°–35°C and the rectal temperature rose above 37.2°C. The threshold rectal temperature for sweating fell during the 10 days after birth. Foster et al. (1969) could not detect sweating in infants of less than 210 days postconceptual age, even when rectal temperature rose as high as 37.8°C. In full-term babies, 414 active sweat glands per square centimeter were found on the thigh, which was 6½ times the number found in adults. The mean maximum sweating rate on chemical stimulation, however, was only 2.4 nl per gland per minute, three times lower than the maximum rate found in the adult.

Circulation

The other important thermoregulatory response to heat is the redistribution of blood in the circulation. The transfer of metabolic heat from the deep tissues to the skin, where it is lost by evaporation, depends on skin blood flow, which under hot conditions is increased relative to other organ blood flows. The early stages of acclimatization to heat are marked by an inadequate cardiovascular response. There is a considerably increased vascular volume relative to blood volume because of widespread peripheral vasodilatation.

The cardiovascular inadequacy of unacclimatized man results from the high skin blood flow, which leads to impaired circulation in the brain, working muscles, and other organs. The overall blood flow to the skin ranges from 0.16 liters m^{-2} min^{-1} in a nude resting man at 28°C to 2.6 liters m^{-2} min^{-1} in a very hot environment. An acclimatized man working for 6 hours at a metabolic rate of 220 W m^{-2} at 50°C with 18 percent relative humidity can maintain thermal equilibrium with a total skin blood flow of 1.2 liters m^{-2} min^{-1} (Robinson, 1963).

Blood flow to the hands and feet is increased under hot conditions by the release of vasoconstrictor tone. Blood flow to the skin of the forearm, however, is increased in the heat by active vasodilatation under nervous control (Chapter 5). Robinson (1963) states that vasodilatation in the hand begins at an environmental temperature of 22°C (although the critical temperature is about 28°C) and occurs in waves as the temperature rises. Vasodilatation of the hand is also induced by warming areas of skin elsewhere on the body. Local warming of the hand then increases vasodilatation further. Vasodilatation in the hand therefore begins at an environmental temperature below the critical level. Between 18°C and 25°C, the vessels of the arms and hands dilate, and then, up to 30°C, the legs and feet show vasodilatation, with a maximum above 31°–

32°C. Measured blood flows per 100 ml of tissue in the foot have ranged from less than 1 ml min^{-1} in the cold to more than 16 ml min^{-1} under hot conditions.

The considerable increase in blood flow through the skin under hot conditions at first produces cardiovascular disturbance. Cardiovascular stability is regained during acclimatization largely through two compensations: vasoconstriction elsewhere than in the skin, and an increased blood volume. Compensatory vasoconstriction in the viscera is illustrated in resting man at 50°C by the reduction in renal blood flow to 60–75 percent of the flow found in a cool environment. Exercise in the heat reduces renal blood flow to 40–50 percent of control values, and dehydration brings about a further decrease.

The rate of blood flow in the skin has the chief influence on the internal conductance of the body; the higher the blood flow and the conductance, the greater the rate of transfer of metabolic heat from the tissues to the skin for each degree centigrade difference. An acclimatized man working under conditions of extreme heat stress can conduct metabolic heat to the skin at a maximal rate of about 90 W m^{-2} per °C temperature difference between rectal and skin temperatures; this coefficient is more than twice that in a man at rest, probably because the rate of blood circulation is higher in an exercising man. These large coefficients are about three times those determined on the same men in corresponding metabolic states in a cool environment, in which cutaneous flow is reduced by vasoconstriction (Robinson, 1949).

Exercise

Shepherd and Webb-Peploe (1970) have discussed the interaction between the blood-flow demands of muscle for activity and of skin for heat dissipation when exercise is performed in the heat. In a comfort-

able environment, the cardiac output is determined largely by metabolic changes in the
active muscle that cause vasodilatation in
the active tissues and vasoconstriction elsewhere. In the heat, skin blood flow must
also be increased. When identical levels of
working in hot and comfortable environments are compared, however, the cardiac
output is not larger in the heat. Because it
can be concluded that skin blood flow is
greater under hot conditions, then either less
blood goes to the active muscles or, what
appears to be the case, less goes to other
organs. It has been demonstrated that renal
and hepatic blood flow shows greater reduction during exercise in the heat than under
comfortable conditions.

The maximal capacity for work in the
heat is reduced because the maximal heart
rate and maximal decrement in visceral
blood flow are reached at lower levels of
work than in a cooler environment. Heart
rate is a criterion for the limitation of heat
tolerance; a reasonable limit for the heart
rate is 100–110 beats per minute while the
subject is sitting, and 120–130 while working. Higher rates may be borne without
undue disturbance for shorter periods, however (Belding, 1970). At submaximal work
levels under hot conditions, the same amount
of blood goes to the active muscles, more to
the skin, and less to the internal organs than
in a comfortable environment. There is in-
sufficient cardiac output to compensate for
dilatation of skin vessels in the heat and the
blood pressure falls. This leads reflexly to
more powerful constriction of the renal and
splanchnic vessels, with the result that the
visceral vessels are maximally constricted
at a lower work load in heat than under
comfortable conditions.

The rate of sweating in man increases
in a constant environment as the metabolic
rate in work increases, in addition to the response to an externally imposed heat stress.
Both rectal temperature and skin temperature appear to be involved in the regulation
of sweating in working men (Robinson,

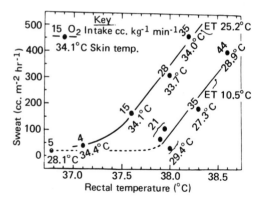

Fig. 10–2. Relation of rate of sweating to
increasing rectal temperature. The increments
in rectal temperature were produced by increasing intensities of work as indicated by O_2 intake (numbers above points) of the subject.
Increasing work did not affect skin temperature
(numbers below points). ET is effective temperature (Robinson, 1949). In *Physiology of
Heat Regulation and the Science of Clothing.*
L. H. Newburgh, Ed. New York: W. B. Saunders, p. 212.

1949). Figure 10–2 shows the relation of
sweating to the rise in rectal temperature
produced by increasing intensities of work.
Oxygen consumption rates vary from 4 ml
kg^{-1} min^{-1} at rest to 44 ml kg^{-1} min^{-1}
when walking on a treadmill at 7.3 km hr^{-1}
up a 9 percent gradient, at two effective temperatures of 10.5°C and 25.2°C. The skin
temperature at each effective temperature is
the same at all levels of work, and at each
skin temperature the rectal temperature and
the rate of sweating increase as the work and
metabolic rate increase. At the same rectal
temperature, for example, 38°C, both the
rate of sweating and the skin temperature
are markedly elevated at the higher effective
temperature. In experiments of this sort,
maximal rates of sweating of 1.3 kg m^{-2}
hr^{-1} have been observed, similar to the maximal rates found by Kerslake and Brebner
(1970) in resting subjects in a heated water
bath.

The heat loss increases when a man
works in the heat, evaporative loss account-

ing for the increase, until a new equilibrium is reached. The rectal temperature also rises and reaches a steady state that corresponds to the rate of working and not to the environmental temperature. However, the skin temperature does not change when the rate of work is increased provided that the environmental temperature remains constant (see Fig. 10–2). When work ceases, the rectal temperature slowly returns to the original level. If heat stress is too severe, an equilibrium is not reached and the body temperature continues to rise. Any combined stress of heat and work that elevates a man's rectal temperature to about 38.8°C within 2 hours results, if continued, in further rises in rectal temperature and exhaustion within the next 4 hours (Robinson, 1949).

Women appear to be affected more adversely than men by short-term exposure to heat stress or to work in the heat; this may be partly because women sweat less than men in severe heat. However, body temperature and circulatory reactions after acclimatization are similar in both men and women. This suggests that unacclimatized women are further from acclimatization than unacclimatized men, possibly because of generally lower levels of activity (Chaffee and Roberts, 1971).

Blood Volume

There is an increase in blood volume in the early days of acclimatization to heat, but this appears to be a temporary phenomenon (Leithead and Lind, 1964). Dehydration leads to a reduction in plasma water proportionately greater than that in total body water. If the subject is not well hydrated under hot conditions, the consequent dehydration prevents the adaptive increase in blood volume, leading to cardiovascular insufficiency and lack of tolerance to heat.

Heat Stress

Many investigations have attempted to produce a reliable measurement of the degree of stress produced by a hot environment. An objective estimate is highly desirable in a situation that is so much open to subjective interpretation, and one such index of heat stress has been put forward by Hatch (1963), from the balance of heat production and heat loss:

$$M + H_R + H_C = H_E$$

where M = metabolic rate
H_R = heat loss or gain by radiation
H_C = heat loss or gain by convection
H_E = heat loss by evaporation

This equation has been discussed in Chapter 2. Hatch analyzes the position of a man in a hot environment in terms of the limitations of blood flow to the skin, heat transfer between blood and skin, and the rate of sweating and evaporation from the skin surface. From this analysis, he suggests the ratio of cutaneous blood flow to cardiac output as a single index of physiological strain, and the rate of sweating as a measurement of heat stress. The strain is thus a measure of the physiological response; as acclimatization progresses, the strain declines markedly. The exposure of unacclimatized men to heat leads in the early stages to marked strain, and the diminution of blood supply to the brain can lead to fainting. Stress, in contrast, is determined by the environment acting on the individual. In this instance, it is indicated by the cooling power required, which is given by the sweating rate. Sweating does not add directly to the physiological cost of heat exposure, although serious overtaxing can lead to failure of the sweating mechanism.

If the stress and strain referred to here are to be really analogous to the stress and strain in the physical example of a weight (stress) acting on a spring to produce a lengthening (strain), the measure of heat stress must be solely a function of the environment and independent of the organism. The use of rate of sweating as a measure of stress means that this is not the case. A response on the part of the organism (sweating) is used to translate the total environmental effect into a measure of stress, and then another response of the organism (the ratio of cutaneous blood flow to cardiac output) is used as a measure of strain. It is clearly necessary to use the organism to measure strain, because strain occurs in the organism. To use the organism also to measure the stress is, in terms of the strict analogy, inadmissible. In practice, however, this measurement of stress is reasonable because the organism can more readily integrate the total effect of the environment than can any purely physical measurements. In commenting on this problem, Kerslake (1972) says:

If heat stress can indeed be expressed independently of physiological responses, and so be defined purely in terms of the environment and clothing, it follows that families of equivalent environments (i.e. imposing the same heat stress) must be the same for all subjects. The strain induced in subject A by heat stress X may be different from that induced in subject B by the same stress, but all environments inducing this strain in subject A must also induce the equivalent strain in subject B (by courtesy of Cambridge University Press).

The several components of the environment are weighted differently for different individuals in terms of their relative effects. This is illustrated for different species in the markedly different weightings attached to dry bulb and wet bulb temperatures for the effects of hot environments in man, cattle, and the pig (see Chapter 9). When man and the pig are exposed to high temperatures, man has a high sweat rate, indicating "stress" in terms of the Hatch index, and the pig has a very low sweat rate, which quite incorrectly indicates a very low "stress" for the same environment. Both organisms have high skin blood flows and so

both indicate high "strain." Kerslake, commenting on the same problem, considers the case of a nonsweating man and concludes that in divergent cases the single-number type of heat stress index and the analogy of stress and strain do not work. The problem of individual variation arises here, different sweating rates in different individuals indicating apparent differences in stress in the same environment. This includes the paradoxical result that as an individual becomes acclimatized to heat and so increases his sweating rate, he apparently is being exposed to a greater heat stress, although his actual tolerance of the hot environment has increased. These limitations of the concept of stress and strain in the heat should be borne in mind when the various "indices of heat" are considered.

Several indices of heat have been developed to describe the stress imposed by a hot environment (Leithead and Lind, 1964). One of the earliest is the wet bulb temperature, used by J. S. Haldane (1905) to assess the effect of high air temperature on man. He concludes that the upper limit of wet bulb that can prevail without a rise in body temperature is 31°C with the subject clothed and at rest in still air, 34°C at an air movement of 50 m min^{-1} and 25°C during the performance of moderate work in still air. These values are still generally acceptable.

Other indices have involved the deep body temperature, heart rate, and such other factors as skin temperature and sweating. The "index of physiological effect" involves all four factors; it is a multiple-response index (Robinson et al., 1945), and consequently might be expected to yield a result that is not so subject to variation as the measurement of a single response. The index was developed by making measurements of rectal and skin temperatures, rate of sweating, and heart rate in well-acclimatized subjects. The four responses were weighted equally, and the lines of constant physiological strain so derived were plotted on the psychrometric chart.

Another index is the "predicted 4-hour

sweat rate" (P4SR) of McArdle et al. (1947), described by Macpherson (1960), which takes account only of the rate of sweating as an indication of heat stress. The effects of air temperature, radiant temperature, humidity, air movement, and rate of working are assessed in two sets of clothing, shorts and overalls. The heat index is read from a nomogram constructed empirically from observations, of 4 hours duration each, made on naval ratings. The nomogram is entered with the globe temperature and a modified wet bulb temperature, giving a basic 4-hour sweat rate. The P4SR is then found by adding to the basic rate amounts that depend on the metabolic rate and clothing. The nomogram is arranged to underestimate hot–dry conditions compared with hot–wet, and to overestimate rate of sweating under severe conditons.

Effective temperature scales have become the best known measures of heat stress, however, and these, together with other systems, have been discussed recently by Belding (1970). The scales originated by the assignment of equivalent effective temperatures to combinations of conditions, each combination producing an equivalent thermal sensation, with particular attention to comfort limits but also extending to hot and cold zones. Several modifications of these scales have been introduced to take account of factors that are under- or overrepresented in the original scales. Modifications for radiant heat load include the "corrected effective temperature" and the "wet bulb : globe temperature index" (WBGT) (see Kerslake, 1972). The WBGT requires three readings: standard black globe thermometer (T_g), shaded dry bulb (T_a), and wet bulb without artificial ventilation (T'_{wb}).

The index is then given by:

$$\text{WBGT} = 0.7T'_{wb} + 0.2T_g + 0.1T_a$$

If the normal wet bulb temperature, that is, the temperature of a forcibly ventilated wet bulb not exposed to radiation, T_{wb}, is used:

$$\text{WBGT} = 0.7T_{wb} + 0.3T_g$$

The WBGT has been valuable in reducing heat casualties during army training; its particular value, coupled with its simplicity, is that it indicates conditions that may cause casualties through heat illness. Its application is therefore particularly appropriate where heat stress reaches a critical level.

Some of the more recent attempts to define the thermal stress imposed on man by the environment have been based on the quantitative assessment of heat exchange through the different channels. Particular emphasis has been placed on evaporative loss from the skin because man can sweat profusely and so lose heat at a rate equivalent to 20 times the resting metabolism. The "heat stress index" (Belding and Hatch, 1955) is based on the ratio of the total evaporative heat loss required, E_{req}, to the total available evaporative heat loss potential, E_{max}. The ratio E_{req}/E_{max} has a value of unity when the evaporative loss is at the limit. At lower values, conditions are less demanding and there is correspondence of the ratio with results obtained by the index of physiological effect (Robinson et al., 1945). E_{req} can be calculated from the sum of the metabolic heat production plus the radiant and convective heat loads. When this difference exceeds E_{max} the difference can be used to predict tolerance time, defined as the time taken for body temperature to rise by 1 °C. This is taken as $60/(E_{req} - E_{max})$, because a heat storage increase of 60 kcal, with a specific heat of 0.83, gives a rise in temperature of 1 °C in a man weighing 72 kg.

Another index involving E_{req} and E_{max} has been developed by Givoni. It is described by Kerslake (1972), who has recently given an extensive treatment of the subject of heat stress and indices used to indicate the intensity of heat stress. Kerslake prefers Givoni's "index of thermal stress" to the heat stress index of Belding and Hatch (1955) because the former makes predictions that accord with both theoretical expectation and practical experience and its structure allows application to various clothing assemblies. Givoni's index covers a wide range of environments and clothing. The P4SR is accurate and valuable in practice but is limited by its empirical nature, and it makes no allowance for sunlight. However, because in practice the precision of a heat stress index should be matched to the situation in which it is used, Kerslake considers that something like the WBGT may be the most suitable index for many purposes.

Heat Tolerance

Physical fitness by itself does not provide tolerance of heat. There is considerable variation between individuals in respect of their tolerance of hot conditions. Wyndham (1970) has discussed this variation with particular reference to Bantu workers in the gold mines of South Africa. The application of methods of heat acclimatization in this industry has been most successful in protecting workers from excessive heat (Fox, 1974). Wyndham has examined the distribution of body temperature in samples of upwards of 100 men, either acclimatized or unacclimatized, under standard conditions of work and environment and with wet bulb temperatures between 30°C and 33°C. He has found the distribution to be skewed toward the higher body temperatures, with men in the skew part of the curve more heat intolerant than others.

A number of factors are associated with intolerance to heat. The main factor is the maximum oxygen intake; men with low maximum oxygen intakes develop higher body temperatures in the heat and consequently show less heat tolerance. Other factors associated with intolerance are previous work in cool conditions and overweight. The prediction of intolerance to heat is improved if all three factors are used in classification. Seventy-five percent of men with adverse scores from the combined factors and only 8 percent of men with good scores are heat intolerant, so that the chances of misplacement arising from selection made on this basis are relatively small.

How well a man can perform tasks under conditions of graded high temperatures depends on his degree of acclimatization. Men acclimatized to the heat and stripped to the waist become less efficient in a variety of tasks when the effective temperature rises above about 30°C, whereas the performance of unacclimatized and clothed men deteriorates at about 10°C lower (Pepler, 1963).

The lengths of time for which men could work safely at high temperatures were investigated by Bell et al. (1971). Their subjects were 87 fit, unacclimatized young men dressed in overalls who worked continuously at the rate of 310 W at dry bulb/wet bulb combinations ranging from 37.0°/30.0°C to 83.4°/41.2°C, with air movement of 0.76 or 1.02 m sec^{-1}. The relation between time taken to imminent heat collapse and environmental severity was calculated and tables were drawn up giving durations of safe exposure for 75, 90, 95, or 99 percent of the subjects. Imminent heat collapse was assessed on the criteria of (a) a high and rapidly rising body temperature above 39°C and a pulse that was irregular or above 200 per minute, (b) the general appearance of the subject and his ability to work, and (c) the subject's own feeling of exhaustion. Examples from the tables of safe duration for exposure to 45°/35°C are 37 minutes for 75 percent of subjects, 31 minutes for 90 percent, 28 minutes for 95 percent, and 23 minutes for 99 percent.

The severity of hot conditions for prolonged and intermittent exposure to heat has been subdivided into three grades (Lind, 1963). Intolerable situations are those in which only short exposure leads to fainting or other effects and in which thermal man–environment equilibrium cannot be established, as in fire-fighting emergencies. The just tolerable situation is that in which equilibrium is established at the limits of thermoregulatory capacity, as in certain industrial or military situations in which only intermittent exposure can be permitted. Dehydration is the principal danger in the just tolerable situation, because sweat losses are so high that drinking cannot be expected to make good the water deficit; it is therefore undesirable to prolong such exposures beyond about 4 hours. Easily tolerable situations are those in which continuous exposure is accompanied by thermal equilibrium without undue physiological strain, as in some everyday industrial work. In fit individuals, the time for which an exposure can be tolerated is usually related to the rate and amount of heat storage in the body (Belding, 1967).

The sweating rate of people indigenous to a hot climate is sometimes less than that of Europeans acclimatized to the same conditions (Edholm, 1972). An investigation into the physiological reactions of different groups living in the same areas has been carried out by Strydom and Wyndham (1963). They have measured responses to a work rate of 1 liter of oxygen consumption per minute performed in a standard hot environment and have concluded that there is little difference in heat tolerance between different groups, provided that the subjects have been active at similar levels in similar environments.

Heat Disorders

Illness or disorders associated with heat are produced by metabolic and environmental heat that together constitute an excessive load on the body. The clinical effects arise not only from the failure of thermoregulation, but also from its success, as in the loss of water and electrolytes in sweat. Syncope may result from cutaneous vasodilatation in response to heat in the unacclimatized man, or it may be caused by the circulatory insufficiency that occurs in salt depletion. Heat exhaustion may or may not be accompanied by a rise in body temperature.

Leithead and Lind (1964) refer to these characteristics and describe the classification and incidence of heat disorders; their text should be consulted for a full account.

1. Disorders complicating thermoregulation. These include:
   a. Heat syncope. This is heat collapse occurring in the absence of observable depletion of water or salt, resulting in giddiness, acute fatigue, or loss of consciousness.
   b. Heat exhaustion related to depletion of water or salt. Water depletion is associated with thirst and pyrexia, leading eventually to delirium and death, whereas salt depletion is associated with nausea, vomiting, giddiness, muscle cramps (the well known miner's cramp), and eventually circulatory failure.
   c. Prickly heat. This is a skin condition associated with prolonged wetting of the skin by sweat and characterized by a prickling sensation when the patient is sweating.
2. Disorders resulting from failure of thermoregulation. These are heat stroke and heat hyperpyrexia. Heat stroke comes on suddenly following exposure to a hot environment, with a high body temperature, absence of sweating, and disturbances of the nervous system. It is frequently fatal. In heat hyperpyrexia, the patient is conscious and may be sweating; the rectal temperature, although high, is usually lower than in heat stroke.
3. Psychological effects of heat. These are apathy, fatigue, and poorer performance of skilled tasks; willingness to work is reduced rather than the capacity to work.

Thermal Comfort

A thermal balance involving man's heat production and his exchanges of heat with the surroundings can be attained over a wide range of environmental conditions. The achievement of such a balance, however, does not necessarily imply that the individual is in thermal comfort.

Fanger (1970) has found that fairly narrow intervals of skin temperature and rate of sweat secretion correspond to thermal comfort. Results from 183 college students, who expressed their degree of thermal comfort subjectively while at different levels of activity, indicated that for acceptable thermal comfort:

$$T_s = 35.7 - 0.032H \qquad (10\text{--}1)$$

where T_s = mean skin temperature (°C)
and H = heat production (kcal m^{-2} hr^{-1})

$$E = 0.42(H - 50) \qquad (10\text{--}2)$$

where E is the rate of evaporative heat loss by sweating (kcal hr^{-1}) for rates of heat production between 50 and 150 kcal m^{-2}hr^{-1}.

The mean skin temperature for constant comfort decreases as activity increases: at $H = 50$ kcal m^{-2}·hr^{-1} (58 W m^{-2}), $T_s = 34$°C, whereas at H = 150 kcal m^{-2}·hr^{-1} (174 W m^{-2}), $T_s = 31$°C. The rate of sweat secretion is zero for comfort under sedentary conditions and then increases as activity increases. Equations (10–1) and (10–2) can be incorporated in the heat balance equation for man to give a rather complicated expression relating a function of activity to a function of clothing and to environmental variables. This allows the calculation of all combinations of air temperature, air humidity, mean radiant temperature, and air velocity that give rise to optimal comfort conditions for persons of the particular group employed. In practice, it is simpler to use diagrams instead of the "comfort equation," and Fanger (1970) gives a number of these for different conditions of clothing (nude, light, medium, and heavy) and activity (sedentary, medium, and high).

A set of such diagrams for persons with medium clothing (1 clo) is reproduced in Fig. 10–3 (A–F), giving the combination of air and mean radiant temperatures and air velocity and the relation to wet bulb temperature for three levels of activity. The lines on the graphs are "comfort lines." The comfort lines cross each other (A and B) when the air temperature is equal to the mean temperature of the outer surface of the clothed body, because at this point the convective heat transfer is zero independently of the air velocity. To the left of the crossing point, surface temperature is higher than air temperature, and a rise in air velocity requires a rise in air temperature for thermal comfort. To the right of the crossing point, the air temperature is higher than the surface temperature. Therefore, heat is being transferred to the body, and an increase in air velocity needs a fall in air temperature for the same degree of comfort.

Figures 10–3D, E, and F show that the influence of humidity on thermal comfort is not very large. A change from dry air to saturated air is compensated for by a fall in temperature of 1.5–3°C. This applies only at thermal comfort; at high temperatures the humidity influences the degree of discomfort to a considerable degree.

Fig. 10–3. (A)–(C) Comfort lines (air temperature versus mean radiant temperature with relative air velocity as parameter) for persons with medium clothing at three different activity levels: (A) sedentary, (B) medium activity, and (C) high activity. t_{mrt} = mean radiant temperature, t_a = air temperature. (D)–(F) Comfort lines (ambient temperature versus wet bulb temperature with relative air velocity as parameter) for persons with medium clothing at three different activity levels: (D) sedentary, (E) medium activity, (F) high activity. RH = relative humidity (Fanger, 1970. In *Physiological and Behavioral Temperature Regulation*, J. D. Hardy, A. P. Gagge, and J. A. J. Stolwijk, Eds., pp. 152–176. Courtesy of Charles C Thomas, publisher, Springfield, Illinois).

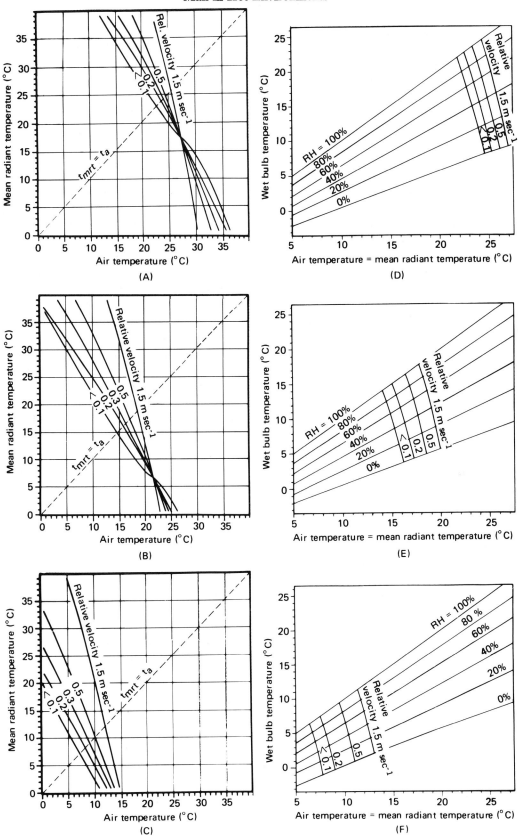

Clothing

The world has been divided into seven "clothing zones" by Siple (1949):

1. Minimum clothing: humid tropical and jungle
2. Hot dry clothing: desert
3. One-layer clothing: subtropical
4. Two-layer clothing: temperate cool winter
5. Three-layer clothing: temperate cold winter
6. Four-layer maximum clothing: subarctic winter
7. Extreme cold: arctic winter

Zones 1 and 2 are those in which man is exposed to hot environments. In zone 3, thermoregulation is maintained with minimum physiological control, and in zones 4, 5, 6, and 7 protection against cold is required to varying degrees.

Zones 1 and 2 are the ones particularly relevant to this text. Regions in which minimum clothing is used (zone 1) are the humid, wet tropical areas, which have average temperatures of between 20°C and 30°C. The peak of radiation intensity occurs at noon, but shelter is provided by vegetation and cloud. Wind velocities are often very low (except for violent storms), averaging 1.5–2.5 m sec^{-1} in the open and less than 0.5 m sec^{-1} in dense vegetation. Because air movement influences both convective and evaporative heat transfer, its absence in a hot humid environment leads to decreased heat dissipation and increased discomfort. Temperatures during the day do not usually rise much above about 33°C and at night do not often drop below 15°–20°C. Daytime relative humidity is 50–75 percent and at night the humidity rises to 100 percent.

In this zone, the need for clothing, excluding cultural considerations, is only to provide protection from strong sunlight and from insects and other damaging material. Apart from these limitations, the naked state is preferable. The design of headgear should allow for an air space between the head and the hat, both to reduce a conductive heat load and to increase the likelihood of heat dissipation consequent on any air movement from a breeze or produced by activity.

The situation is quite different in the desert (zone 2). A hot day in the desert may have a temperature of 40°–45°C, or even higher, with a relative humidity of 10 percent, whereas a hot day in the wet tropics may have a temperature of 33°–35°C, with a relative humidity of 85 percent. In the desert, clothing is required for protection against the heat because environmental temperatures rise above body temperature. There are clear skies, low humidity, and cool nights. Suitable clothing should therefore protect against sun and high temperature during the day, while allowing the evaporation of sweat, and serve also as protection against cold at night.

Radiation, both solar and reradiation from the surroundings, is intense during the day, and dry winds at high air temperatures burn and desiccate. Heat transfer by radiation, convection, and conduction is therefore inward from the environment and constitutes a heat load. This is added to the metabolic heat load and must be dissipated entirely by evaporative heat transfer. The total heat load is equivalent to that of strenuous exercise. Night temperatures average 15°–20°C, although on occasion these drop below the freezing point, and the 24-hourly fluctuation in temperature can be very marked, up to 30°C or even more. Wind velocities are commonly 5–8 m·sec^{-1} and may average 10–15 m·sec^{-1}. The average desert humidity is 15–20 mbar vapor pressure and does not generally rise above 25–30 mbar; at an air temperature of 45°C this produces a relative humidity of 20–30 percent. In the driest deserts the vapor pressure may fall below 1 mbar. (See also p. 124.)

Under hot desert conditions, clothing must insulate against radiant, convective, and conductive heat transfer from the environment. It must also allow the vaporization of sweat while controlling air movement, however, for when the air temperature is above body temperature, increasing air movement at the body surface leads to an increased heat load. Adequate ventilation is therefore necessary if evaporation is to be maintained.

The voluminous, loosely worn thick wool or mohair robe of native desert people is admirably suited to this purpose, although such clothing is not feasible for those who work in desert conditions. The thickness of the robe acts as insulation against heat gain during the day and as insulation against heat loss during the night. During the day its loose folds allow ventilation at the body surface, controlling the strong hot winds impinging on the outside of the robe. Evaporative transfer is helped further as water vapor is removed from the air next to the skin by the turbulent air movements produced by walking and other activity. If the robe is wetted, evaporation in the substance of the robe cools the robe and not the skin, but this has the effect of dissipating the incident heat load and of assisting the "air conditioning" of the space between the robe and the body. Evaporation from the clothing is always less effective than evaporation from the skin in removing heat from the body because the whole of the air-cooling effect of the wet clothing is never entirely used for body cooling; some is always lost to the environment.

The surface of the robe is dark, so both short-wave and long-wave radiation are absorbed (Chapter 2). A light-colored robe allows reflection of some of the incident short-wave radiation, producing a rather lower temperature at the surface of the robe and leaving a smaller quantity of heat to be lost by reradiation or convection. One reason a dark robe is used may be that it is possible to make the material into an opaque, densely woven sheet, whereas a material lighter in color may allow some translucence, with consequent radiant effects directly on the skin surface. The fully absorbent dark, but opaque, material may then be preferable to a partially reflective, but partially translucent, material. To a large extent, the dark clothing is fortuitous; it is cheaper and most

clothing as worn by desert people quickly becomes dirty.

Under hot desert conditions clothing reduces the rate of heat gain from the environment, and there is a correspondingly lower rate of sweating in clothed men than in nude men. This is true particularly for resting man, where an increased heat gain of more than 100 W can be associated with lack of clothing. Experiment has shown that the effect of clothing is to reduce heat gain because oxygen consumption and the rate of change of heat storage are not influenced by clothing. During exercise, however, closely-fitting clothing may hinder the evaporation of sweat, so that evaporative cooling is incomplete. This is more likely to be the case when the ambient humidity is rather higher than the lower levels usually found in the desert, although under dry indoor experimental conditions higher sweating rates have been found in men walking in poplin uniforms than in men walking in shorts.

Robinson (1949) has found that cloth-

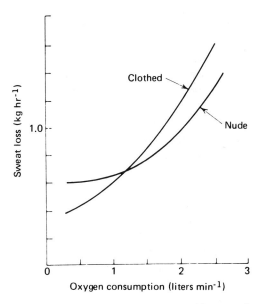

Fig. 10–4. The effect of clothing on the sweat loss of subjects in the desert. At low work rates, the clothing is beneficial because it acts as a radiation screen. At higher work rates this effect is overridden by the restriction of evaporation (from Adolph, 1949).

ing reduces heat absorption by resting men in the summer sun, but the advantage of clothing disappears at a metabolic rate of 280 W m^{-2}. At higher rates of work, moreover, clothing increases the evaporative requirements. Figure 10–4 illustrates this; clothing is beneficial at low metabolic rates but becomes an embarrassment at higher rates, when evaporation is impeded enough to outweigh the screen to radiation provided by the clothing. Although clothing is preferable both for comfort and for reducing heat load when the sun shines on the resting individual, it may be a relative disadvantage under some conditions of exercise.

The feet require protection from the hot ground. This can be achieved by sandals, provided that the upper surfaces of the feet are protected from sunburn. Head protection in hot deserts usually takes the form of a turban or cloth, which offers some insulation and some reflection of incident radiation and which is not as likely to be blown off in a strong wind as a helmet with a brim. However, a well-ventilated helmet reduces sweat rate by 55 gm hr^{-1} (about 38 W equivalent) in a man sitting or walking in the sun, in addition to shading the eyes and keeping the top of the head about 6°C cooler than a bare head (Robinson, 1949). The principles of ventilation, wind penetration, and radiation characteristics of clothing have been discussed in relation to evaporative heat loss by Kerslake (1972).

References

* An asterisk indicates a review, or an article taken from a book containing other relevant material.

Adair, E. R., Casby, J. U., and Stolwijk, J. A. J. (1970). Behavioral temperature regulation in the squirrel monkey: Changes induced by shifts in hypothalamic temperature. *J. Comp. Physiol. Psychol.* **72:** 17–27.

*Adolph, E. F. (1947). *Physiology of Man in the Desert.* New York: Interscience.

*Adolph, E. F. (1949). Desert. In *Physiology of Heat Regulation and the Science of Clothing.* L. H. Newburgh, Ed. Philadelphia: Saunders, pp. 330–338.

Alexander, G. (1961). Temperature regulation in the new-born lamb. II. A climatic respiration chamber for the study of thermoregulation. *Aust. J. Agric. Res.* **12:** 1139–1151.

*Alexander, G. (1974). Heat loss from sheep. In *Heat Loss from Animals and Man: Assessment and Control*, J. L. Monteith and L. E. Mount, Eds. London: Butterworths.

Allen, T. E., and Bligh, J. (1969). A comparative study of the temporal patterns of cutaneous water vapour loss from some domesticated mammals with epitrichial sweat glands. *Comp. Biochem. Physiol.* **31:** 347–363.

*Andersson, B. (1964). Hypothalamic temperature and thyroid activity. In *Brain–Thyroid Relationships.* Ciba Found. Study Group **18:** 35–50.

*Andersson, B., Gale, C. C., and Hökfelt, B. (1964). Studies of the interaction between neural and hormonal mechanisms in the regulation of body temperature. In *Major Problems in Neuroendocrinology*, E. Bajusz and G. Jasmin, Eds. Basel and New York: Karger, pp. 42–61.

Andersson, B., Gale, C. C., Hökfelt, B., and Larsson, B. (1965). Acute and chronic effects of preoptic lesions. *Acta Physiol. Scand.* **65:** 45–60.

Andersson, B., Grant, R., and Larsson, S. (1956). Central control of heat loss mechanisms in the goat. *Acta Physiol. Scand.* **37:** 261–280.

Aoki, T. (1955). Stimulation of the sweat glands in the hairy skin of the dog by adrenaline, noradrenaline, acetylcholine mecholyl and pilocarpine. *J. Invest. Derm.* **24:** 545–556.

Aoki, T., and Wada, M. (1951). Functional activity of the sweat glands on the hairy skin of the dog. *Science* **114:** 123–127.

Armsby, H. P., and Fries, J. A. (1903). The available energy of "Timothy" hay. U.S. Dept. of Agriculture Bull. 51.

Aschoff, J., and Wever, R. (1957). Durchblulungsmessung an menschlichen Extremität. *Verhandl. Deut. Ges. Kreislaufforsch* **23:** 375–380.

Aschoff, J., and Wever, R. (1958). Kern und Schale im Wärmehaushalt des Menechen. *Naturwissenschaften* **45:** 477–485.

*Atkins, E. (1960). Pathogenesis of fever. *Physiol. Rev.* **40:** 580–648.

Atwater, W. O., and Benedict, F. G. (1905). A respiration calorimeter with appliances for the direct determination of oxygen. Carnegie Institute, Washington, Publ. No. 42.

Auget, A., and Lefèvre, J. (1929). Nouvelle chambre calorimetrique du laboratoire de bioenérgetique. *Compt. Rend. Hebd. Seanc. Acad. Sci. (Paris)* **100:** 251–253.

Baldwin, B. A. (1968). Behavioural thermoregulation in mice. *Physiol. Behav.* **3:** 401–407.

Baldwin, B. A., and Ingram, D. L. (1967a). The effect of heating and cooling the hypothalamus on behavioural thermoregulation in the pig. *J. Physiol. (London)* **191:** 375–392.

Baldwin, B. A., and Ingram, D. L. (1967b). Behavioural thermoregulation in pigs. *Physiol. Behav.* **2:** 15–21.

Baldwin, B. A., and Ingram, D. L. (1968). The influence of hypothalamic temperature and ambient temperature on thermoregulatory mechanisms in the pig. *J. Physiol. (London)* **198:** 517–529.

Baldwin, B. A., and Lipton, J. M. (1973). Central and peripheral temperatures and EEG changes during behavioural thermoregulation in pigs. *Acta Neurobiol. Exp.* **33:** 433–447.

Banerjee, M. R., Elizondo, R., and Bullard, R. W. (1969). Reflex responses of human sweat glands to different rates of skin cooling. *J. Appl. Physiol.* **26:** 787–792.

Barbour, H. G. (1912). Die Wirkung unmittelbarer Erwärmung und Abkühlung der Wärmezentra auf die Köpertemperatur. *Arch. Exp. Pathol. Pharmakol.* **70:** 1–26.

*Bartholomew, G. A. (1964). Homeostasis in the desert environment. In *Homeostasis and Feedback Mechanisms*, Society for Experimental Biology, Symposium No. 18. London: Cambridge University Press.

Bartholomew, G. A., Hudson, J. W. and Howell, T. R. (1962). Body temperature, oxygen consumption, evaporative water loss and heart rate in the poor-will. *Condor* **64:** 117–125.

Bartholomew, G. A., Lasiewski, R. C., and Crawford, E. C. (1968). Patterns of panting and gular flutter in cormorants, pelicans, owls and doves. *Condor* **70:** 31.

Bartholomew, G. A., and Tucker, V. A. (1963). Control of changes in body temperature, metabolism and circulation by the agamid lizard, *Amphibolurus barbatus*. *Physiol. Zool.* **36:** 199–218.

*Bass, D. E. (1963). Thermoregulatory and circulatory adjustments during acclimatization to heat in man. In *Temperature, Its Measurement and Control in Science and Industry*, Vol. 3, Pt.3, J. D. Hardy, Ed. New York: Reinhold, pp. 299–305.

*Bazett, H. C. (1949). The regulation of body temperature. In *Physiology of Heat Regulation and the Science of Clothing*, L. H. Newburgh, Ed. Philadelphia: Saunders, 109–192.

Beakley, W. R., and Findlay, J. D. (1955). The effect of environmental temperature and humidity on the respiration rate of Ayrshire calves. *J. Agric. Sci. (Cambridge)* **45:** 452–460.

Bedford, T. (1946). *Environmental Warmth and Its Measurement.* Medical Research Council, London: H.M.S.O.

*Belding, H. S. (1967). Resistance to heat in man and other homeothermic animals. In *Thermobiology*, A. H. Rose, Ed. London: Academic Press, pp. 479–510.

*Belding, H. S. (1970). The search for a universal heat stress index. In *Physiological and Behavioral Temperature Regulation*, J. D. Hardy, A. P. Gagge, and J. A. J. Stolwijk, Eds. Springfield, Ill.: Charles C Thomas, pp. 193–202.

Belding, H. S., and Hatch, T. F. (1955). Index for evaluating heat stress in terms of the resulting physiological strain. *Heat. Pip. Air Condit.* **27,** Aug.: 129–136.

Bell, C. R., Crowder, M. J., and Walters, J. D.

(1971). Durations of safe exposure for men at work in high temperature environments. *Ergonomics* **14:** 733–757.

Benzinger, T. H. (1959). On physical heat regulation and the sense of temperature in man. *Proc. Natn. Acad. Sci. U.S.A.* **45:** 645–659.

*Benzinger, T. H. (1969). Heat regulation: Homeostasis of central temperature. *Physiol. Rev.* **49:** 671–759.

*Benzinger, T. H. (1971). Peripheral cold reception and central warm reception, sensory mechanisms of behavioural and autonomic thermostasis. In *Physiological and Behavioral Temperature Regulation*, J. D. Hardy, A. P. Gagge, and J. A. J. Stolwijk, Eds. Springfield, Ill.: Charles C Thomas, Chap. 56.

Benzinger, T. H., Heubscher, R. G., Minard, D., and Kitzinger, C. (1958). Human calorimetry by means of the gradient principle. *J. Appl. Physiol.* **12:** S1–S28.

Benzinger, T. H., and Kitzinger, C. (1949). Direct calorimetry by means of the gradient principle. *Rev. Sci. Instrum.* **20:** 849–860.

*Benzinger, T. H., and Kitzenger, C. (1963). Gradient layer calorimetry and human calorimetry. In *Temperature, Its Measurement and Control in Science and Industry*, Vol. III, Pt. 3, C. M. Hertzfeld and J. D. Hardy, Eds. New York: Reinhold, pp. 87–109.

*Benzinger, T. H., Kitzinger, C., and Pratt, A. W. (1963). The human thermostat. In *Heat*, Vol. 3, Pt. 3, C. M. Hertzfeld and J. D. Hardy, Eds. London and New York: Reinhold, pp. 637–665.

Berde, B. (1948). Nervous control of thermothyrine-A secretion of the thyroid. *Experientia* **4:** 231–232.

*Berde, B. (1951). Wärmeregulation und endokrines System. *Zschr. Vitamin u. Forsch. (Wien)* **4:** 338–376.

Bianca, W. (1959). Acclimatization of calves to a hot dry environment. *J. Agric. Sci. (Cambridge)* **52:** 296–304.

Bianca, W. (1962). Relative importance of dry and wet bulb temperatures in causing heat stress in cattle. *Nature (London)* **195:** 251–252.

*Bianca, W. (1968). Thermoregulation. In *Adaptation of Domestic Animals*, E. S.

E. Hafez, Ed. Philadelphia: Lea and Febiger, pp. 97–118.

Bianca, W., and Findlay, J. D. (1962). The effect of thermally-induced hypernoea on the acid–base status of the blood of calves. *Res. Vet. Sci.* **3:** 38–49.

Blagden, C. (1774). Experiments and observations in an heated room. *Phil. Trans. Roy. Soc.* **65:** 111–123.

Blagden, C. (1775). Further experiments and observations in an heated room. *Phil. Trans. Roy. Soc.* **65:** 484–494.

*Blaxter, K. L. (1967). *The Energy Metabolism of Ruminants*, 2nd ed. Springfield, Ill.: Charles C Thomas.

Blaxter, K. L., Graham, N. McC., Wainman, F. W., and Armstrong, D. G. (1959a). Environmental temperature, energy metabolism and heat regulation in sheep. II. The partition of heat losses in closely clipped sheep. *J. Agric. Sci. (Cambridge)* **52:** 25–40.

Bligh, J. (1957a). A comparison of the temperature of the blood in the pulmonary artery and in the bicarotid trunk of the calf during thermal polypnoea. *J Physiol. (London)* **136:** 404–412.

Bligh, J. (1957b). The initiation of thermal polypnoea in the calf. *J. Physiol. (London)* **136:** 413–419.

Bligh, J. (1961). The synchronous discharge of apocrine sweat glands of the Welsh mountain sheep. *Nature (London)* **189:** 582–583.

*Bligh, J. (1966). The thermosensitivity of the hypothalamus and thermoregulation in mammals. *Biol. Rev.* **41:** 317–367.

Bligh, J. (1967). A thesis concerning the processes of secretion and discharge of sweat. *Environ. Res.* **1:** 28–45.

*Bligh, J. (1972). Neuronal models of mammalian temperature regulation. In *Essays on Temperature Regulation*, J. Bligh and R. Moore, Eds. Amsterdam and London: North Holland.

*Bligh, J. (1973). *Temperature Regulation in Mammals and Other Vertebrates*. Amsterdam and London: North Holland.

Bligh, J., Cottle, W. H., and Maskrey, M. (1971). Influence of ambient temperature on the thermoregulatory responses to 5-hydroxytryptamine, noradrenaline and acetylcholine injected into the lateral cerebral ventricles of sheep, goats and rabbits. *J. Physiol. (London)* **212**: 377–392.

Bogert, C. M., and Cowles, R. B. (1959). How reptiles regulate their body temperature. *Sci. Amer.* **200**: 105–120.

Bond, T. F., Kelly, C. F., Morrison, S. R., and Pereira, N. (1967). Solar, atmospheric and terrestrial radiation received by shaded and unshaded animals. *Trans. Am. Soc. Agric. Eng.* **10**: 622–625, 627.

Bretz, W. L., and Schmidt-Nielsen, K. (1970). Patterns of air flow in the duck lung. *Fed. Proc.* **29**: 662.

Brockway, J. M., McDonald, J. D., and Pullar, J. D. (1965). Evaporative heat loss mechanisms in sheep. *J. Physiol. (London)* **179**: 554–568.

*Brody, S. (1945). *Bioenergetics and Growth.* New York: Reinhold.

Brook, A. H., and Short, B. F. (1960). Sweating in sheep. *Aust. J. Agric. Res.* **11**: 557–569.

Brooks, J. R., Pipes, G. W., and Ross, C. V. (1962). Effect of temperature on the thyroxine secretion rate of rams. *J. Anim. Sci.* **21**: 414–417.

Buettner, K. (1953). Diffusion of water and water vapour through human skin. *J. Appl. Physiol.* **6**: 229–242.

Bullard, R. W., Dill, D. B., and Yousef, M. K. (1970). Responses of the burro to desert heat stress. *J. Appl. Physiol.* **29**: 159–167.

Burton, A. C. (1935). The average temperature of the tissues of the body. *J. Nutr.* **9**: 261–280.

*Burton, A. C., and Edholm, O. G. (1955). *Man in a Cold Environment.* London: Edward Arnold.

Cabanac, H. P., and Hammel, H. T. (1971). Comportement thermorégulateur du lézard *Tiliqua scincoides*: réponses au froid. *J. Physiol. (Paris)* **63**: 222–225.

Cabanac, M. (1969). Plaisir ou Déplaisir de la Sensation Thermique et Homeothermie. *Physiol. Behav.* **4**: 359–364.

Cabanac, M., Stolwijk, J. A. J., and Hardy, J. D. (1968). Effect of temperature and pyrogens on single unit activity in rabbit's brain stem. *J. Appl. Physiol.* **24**: 645–652.

Calder, W. A., and Schmidt-Nielsen, K. (1966). Evaporative cooling and respiratory alkalosis in the pigeon. *Proc. Natl. Acad. Sci. U.S.* **55**: 750–756.

Calder, W. A., and Schmidt-Nielsen, K. (1967). Temperature regulation and evaporation in the pigeon and the roadrunner. *Am. J. Physiol.* **213**: 883–889.

Cannon, P., and Keatinge, W. R. (1960). The metabolic rate and heat loss of fat and thin men in heat balance in cold and warm water. *J. Physiol. (London)* **154**: 329–344.

Capstick, J. W. (1921). A calorimeter for use with large animals. *J. Agric. Sci (Cambridge)* **11**: 408–431.

Capstick, J. W., and Wood, T. B. (1922). The effect of change of temperature on the basal metabolism of swine. *J. Agric. Sci. (Cambridge)* **12**: 257–268.

Carlisle, H. J. (1966a). Heat intake and hypothalamic temperature during behavioral temperature regulation. *J. Comp. Physiol. Psychol.* **61**: 388–397.

Carlisle, H. J. (1966b). Behavioural significance of hypothalamic temperature-sensitive cells. *Nature (London)* **209**: 1324–1325.

Carlisle, H. J., and Ingram, D. L. (1973). The effects of heating and cooling the spinal cord and hypothalamus on thermoregulatory behaviour in the pig. *J. Physiol. (London)* **231**: 353–364.

*Carlson, L. D., and Hsieh, A. C. L. (1970). *Control of Energy Exchange.* London: Macmillan.

Carlton, P. L., and Marks, R. A. (1958). Cold exposure and heat reinforced operant behavior. *Science* **128**: 1344.

*Chaffee, R. R. J., and Roberts, J. C. (1971). Temperature acclimation in birds and mammals. *Ann. Rev. Physiol.* **33**: 155–202.

Chai, C. Y., and Wang, S. C. (1970). Cardiovascular and respiratory responses from local heating of the medulla oblongata of the cat. *Proc. Soc. Exptl. Biol. Med.* **134**: 763–767.

Chatonnet, J., Cabanac, M., and Mottaz, M. (1964). Les conditions de temperatures cérébrale et cutanée moyenne pour l'apparition de la polypnée thermique chez le chien. *Compt. Rend. Séanc. Soc. Biol.* **158**: 1354–1356.

Chauduri, S., and Sadhu, D. P. (1961). Thyroid activity at higher ambient temperatures. *Nature (London)* **192**: 560–561.

Chowers, I., Hammel, H. T., Eisenman, J., Abrams, R. M., and McCann, S. M. (1966). Comparison of effect of environmental and preoptic heating and pyrogen on plasma cortisol. *Am. J. Physiol.* **210:** 606–610.

*Clarke, K. C. (1967). Insects and temperature. In *Thermobiology*, A. H. Rose, Ed. London: Academic Press, pp. 293–352.

*Cloudsley-Thompson, J. L. (1970). Terrestrial invertebrates. In *Comparative Physiology of Thermoregulation*, G. C. Whittow, Ed. New York and London: Academic Press, pp. 15–70.

*Cloudsley-Thompson, J. L. (1971). *The Temperature and Water Relations of Reptiles.* Watford: Merrow.

*Cloudsley-Thompson, J. L., and Chadwick, M. J. (1964). *Life in Deserts.* Philadelphia: Dufour.

Collins, K. J., Hellmann, K., Jones, R. M., and Lunnon, J. B. (1955). Aldosterone activity in the urine of men exposed to heat. *J. Endocrinol.* **13:** 8P.

Collins, K. J., and Weiner, J. S. (1962). The effect of heat acclimatization on the activity and number of sweat glands: a study on Indians and Europeans. *J. Physiol. (London)* **177:** 16–17P.

*Collins, K. J., and Weiner, J. S. (1968). Endocrinological aspects of exposure to high environmental temperatures. *Physiol. Rev.* **48:** 785–839.

Cooper, K. E., and Kerslake, D. McK. (1954). Some aspects of the reflex control of the cutaneous circulation. In *Peripheral Circulation in Man*, G. E. W. Wolstenholme and J. S. Freeman, Eds. London: Churchill, pp. 143–152.

*Corbit, J. D. (1970). Behavioral thermoregulation of body temperature. In *Physiological and Behavioral Temperature Regulation*, J. D. Hardy, A. P. Gagge, and J. A. J. Stolwijk, Eds. Springfield, Ill.: Charles C Thomas, pp. 777–800.

Cormia, F. E., and Kuykendall, V. (1955). Cytochemical studies of eccrine sweat tubules: cellular differentiation and glycogen content. *J. Invest. Derm.* **24:** 527–535.

Cowles, R. B. (1958). Possible origin of dermal temperature regulation. *Evolution* **12:** 347–357.

Crawford, E. C. (1962). Mechanical aspects of panting in dogs. *J. Appl. Physiol.* **17:** 249–251.

Crawford, E. C., and Schmidt-Nielsen, K. (1967). Temperature regulation and evaporative cooling in the ostrich. *Am. J. Physiol.* **212:** 347–353.

Custance, A. C. (1962). Cycling of sweat gland activity recorded by a new technique. *J. Appl. Physiol.* **17:** 741–742.

*Dawson, T. J. (1972). Thermoregulation in Australian desert kangaroos. In *Comparative Physiology of Desert Animals*, G. M. O. Maloiy, Ed. London: Academic Press, pp. 133–146.

*Dawson, W. R., and Hudson, J. W. (1970). Birds. In *Comparative Physiology of Thermoregulation, Vol. 1: Invertebrates and non-mammalian vertebrates*, G. C. Whittow, Ed. New York: Academic Press, pp. 223–310.

*Dawson, W. R., and Schmidt-Nielsen, K. (1964). Terrestrial animals in dry heat: desert birds. In *Handbook of Physiology, Section 4: Adaptation to Environment*, D. B. Dill, Ed. Washington, D.C.: American Physiological Society, pp. 481–492.

Dawson, W. R., and Templeton, J. R. (1963). Physiological responses to temperature in the lizard, *Crotaphytus collaris. Physiol. Zool.* **36:** 219–236.

Dawson, W. R., and Templeton, J. R. (1966). Physiological responses to temperature in the alligator lizard, *Gerrhonotus multicarinatus. Ecology* **47:** 759–765.

Day, R., and Hardy, J. D. (1942). Respiratory metabolism in infancy and in childhood. 26. A calorimeter for measuring the heat loss of premature infants. *Am. J. Dis. Child.* **63:** 1086–1095.

Deighton, T. (1937). A study of the fasting metabolism of various breeds of hog. III. Metabolism and surface area measurements. *J. Agric. Sci. (Cambridge)* **27:** 317–331.

Dempsey, E. W., and Astwood, E. B. (1943). Determination of the rate of thyroid hormone secretion at various environmental temperatures. *Endocrinology* **32:** 509–518.

De Witt, C. B. (1971). Postural mechanisms in the behavioural thermoregulation of a desert lizard, *Dipsosaurus dorsalis. J. Physiol. (Paris)* **63:** 242–245.

Dill, D. B., Bock, A. V., and Edwards, H. T. (1933). Mechanisms for dissipating heat in man and dog. *Am. J. Physiol.* **104:** 36–43.

Donhoffer, S., Mestyán, G., Obrincsák, E., Pap, T., and Tóth, I. (1953a). The mechanism of the rise in O₂ consumption in hyperthermia. *Acta physiol. hung.* **4:** 63–69.

Donhoffer, S., Mestyán, G., Obrincsák, E., Pap, T., and Tóth, I. (1953b). The thermoregulatory significance of the increase in O₂ consumption elicited by high environmental temperature. *Acta physiol. hung.* **4:** 291–299.

*Edholm, O. G. (1972). The effect in man of acclimatization to heat on water intake, sweat rate and water balance. In *Advances in Climatic Physiology*, S. Ito, K. Ogata, and H. Yoshimura, Eds. Tokyo: Shoin, pp. 144–155.

Edholm, O. G., Fox, R. H., and Macpherson, R. K. (1956). Effect of body heating on circulation in the skin and muscle. *J. Physiol. (London)* **134:** 612–619.

*Edney, E. B. (1957). *The Survival of Animals in Hot Deserts*. Oxford: Oxford University Press.

Edney, E. B., and Barrass, R. (1962). The body temperature of the tsetse fly, *Plossina morsitans* Westwood (Diptera, Muscidae). *J. Insect Physiol.* **8:** 469–481.

*Eisenmann, J. S. (1972). Unit activity studies of thermoreceptive neurons. In *Essays on Temperature Regulation,* J. Bligh and R. E. Moore, Eds. Amsterdam and London: North Holland, pp. 55–69.

Epstein, A. N., and Milestone, R. (1968). Showering as a coolant for rats exposed to heat. *Science* **160:** 895–896.

Evans, C. L., Nisbet, A., and Ross, K. A. (1957). A histological study of the sweat glands of normal and drycoated horses. *J. Comp. Pathol.* **67:** 397–405.

Evans, C. L., and Smith, D. F. G. (1956). Sweating responses in the horse. *Proc. Roy. Soc. B. (London)* **145:** 61–83.

Evans, S. E., and Ingram, D. L. (1974). The significance of deep body temperature in regulating the concentration of thyroxine in the plasma of the pig. *J. Physiol. (London)* **236:** 159–170.

*Fanger, P. O. (1970). Conditions for thermal comfort: introduction of a general comfort equation. In *Physiological and Behavioral Temperature Regulation*, J. D. Hardy, A. P. Gagge, and J. A. J. Stolwijk, Eds. Springfield, Ill.: Charles C Thomas, pp. 152–176.

Feldberg, W., and Myers, R. D. (1964) Temperature changes produced by amines injected into the cerebral ventricles during anaesthesia *J. Physiol. (London)* **175:** 464–478.

*Findlay, J. D. (1954). The climatic physiology of farm animals. *Met. Monogr.* **2:** 19–29.

Findlay, J. D. (1957). The respiratory activity of calves subjected to thermal stress. *J. Physiol. (London)* **136:** 300–309.

Findlay, J. D., and Ingram, D. L. (1961). Brain temperature as a factor in the control of thermal polypnea in the ox (*Bos taurus*). *J. Physiol. (London)* **155:** 72–85.

Findlay, J. D., and Robertshaw, D. (1965). The role of the sympatho-adrenal system in the control of sweating in the ox. *J. Physiol. (London)* **179:** 285–297.

Findlay, J. D., and Thompson, G. E. (1968). The effect of intraventricular injections of noradrenaline, 5-hydroxytryptamine, acetylcholine and tranylcypromine on the ox (*Bos taurus*) at different environmental temperatures. *J. Physiol. (London)* **194:** 809–816.

Findlay, J. D., and Whittow, G. C. (1966). The role of arterial oxygen tension in the respiratory response to localized heating of the hypothalamus and to hyperthermia. *J. Physiol (London)* **186:** 333–346.

Findlay, J. D., and Yang, S. H. (1951). The sweat glands of Ayrshire cattle. *J. Agric. Sci. (Cambridge)* **40:** 126–133.

*Folk, G. E. (1966). *Introduction to Environmental Physiology*. London: Kimpton.

Foster, K. G., Hey, E. N., and Katz, G. (1969). The response of the sweat glands of the new-born baby to thermal stimuli and to intradermal acetylcholine. *J. Physiol. (London)* **203:** 13–29.

*Fox, R. H. (1974). Heat acclimatization and the sweating response. In *Heat Loss from Animals and Man: Assessment and Control*, J. L. Monteith and L. E. Mount, Eds. London: Butterworths, pp. 277–301.

Fox, R. H., Goldsmith, R., Kidd, D. J., and Lewis, G. P. (1961). Bradykinin as a vasodilator in man. *J. Physiol. (London)* **157:** 589–602.

Fox, R. H., and Hilton, S. M. (1958). Brady-kinin formation in human skin as a factor in heat vasodilatation. *J. Physiol (London)* **142:** 219–232.

Fox, R. H., Löfstedt, B. E., Woodward, P. M., Eriksson, E., and Werkstrom, B. (1969). Comparison of thermoregulatory function in men and women. *J. Appl. Physiol.* **26:** 444–453.

Frankel, H. M., and Frascella, D. (1968). Blood respiratory gases, lactate and pyruvate during thermal stress in the chicken. *Proc. Soc. Exp. Biol. Med.* **127:** 997–999.

Frankel, H. M., Hollands, K. G., and Weiss, H. S. (1962). Respiratory and circulatory responses of hyperthermic chickens. *Arch. Int. Physiol. Biochim.* **70:** 555–580.

Frisch, K. (1955). *The Dancing Bees.* London: Methuen.

*Fry, F. E. J. (1967). Responses of vertebrate poikilotherms to temperature. In *Thermobiology*, A. H. Rose, Ed. London: Academic Press, pp. 375–409.

*Fry, F. E. J., and Hochacka, P. W. (1970). Fish. In *Comparative Physiology of Thermoregulation*, Vol. 1, G. C. Whittow, Ed. New York: Academic Press, Chapter 3, pp. 79–130.

Fuhrman, G. J., and Fuhrman, F. A. (1959). Oxygen consumption of animals and tissues as a function of temperature. *J. Gen. Physiol.* **42:** 715–722.

Funk, J. P. (1959). Improved polythene-shielded net radiometer. *J. Sci. Instrum.* **36:** 267–270.

Fusco, M. M., Hardy, J. D., and Hammel, H. T. (1961). Interaction of central and peripheral factors in physiological temperature regulation. *Am. J. Physiol.* **200:** 572–580.

Gagge, A. P. (1940). Standard operative temperature, a generalized temperature scale, applicable to direct and partitional calorimetry. *Am. J. Physiol.* **131:** 93–103.

*Gagge, A. P. (1970). Effective radiant flux, an independent variable that describes thermal radiation on man. In *Physiological and Behavioral Temperature Regulation*, J. D. Hardy, A. P. Gagge, and J. A. J. Stolwijk, Eds. Springfield, Ill.: Charles

C Thomas, pp. 34–45.

Gagge, A. P., Winslow, C.-E. A., and Herrington, L. P. (1938). The influence of clothing on the physiological reactions of the human body to varying environmental temperatures. *Am. J. Physiol.* **124:** 30–50.

*Gale, C. C. (1973). Neuroendocrine aspects of thermoregulation. *Ann. Rev. Physiol.* **35:** 391–430.

Gale, C. C., Matthews, M., and Young, J. (1970). Behavioral thermoregulatory responses to hypothalamic cooling and warming in baboons. *Physiol. Behav.* **5:** 1–6.

Gibbons, J. H., and Landis, E. M. (1932). Vasodilatation in the lower extremities in response to immersing the forearm in warm water. *J. Clin. Invest.* **11:** 1019–1036.

Gisolfi, C., and Robinson, S. (1970). Central and peripheral stimuli regulating sweating during intermittent work in men. *J. Appl. Physiol.* **29:** 761–768.

Goldberg, I. J. L., Richards, R., McFarlane, H., and Harland, W. A. (1964). Thyroid uptake of radioiodine in normal subjects in Jamaica. *J. Clin. Endocrinol. Metab.* **24:** 1178–1181.

Goodman, W. (1944). Air conditioning analysis. New York: MacMillan.

Graham, N. McC., Wainman, F. W., Blaxter, K. L., and Armstrong, D. G. (1959). Environmental temperature, energy metabolism and heat regulation in sheep. 1. Energy metabolism in closely clipped sheep. *J. Agric. Sci. (Cambridge)* **52:**13–24.

Grant, R. T. (1963). Vasodilatation and body warming in the rat. *J. Physiol. (London)* **167:** 311–317.

Grayson, J. (1949). Vascular reactions in the human intestine. *J. Physiol. (London)* **109:** 439–447.

Green, H. D., Howard, W. B., and Kenan, L. F. (1956). Autonomic control of blood flow in the hind paw of the dog. *Am. J. Physiol.* **187:** 469–472.

Greenfield, A. D. M. (1963). The circulation through the skin. In *Handbook of Physiology*, Section 2, Vol. 2. Washington, D.C.: American Physiological Society, pp. 1325–1352.

Guieu, J. D. and Hardy, J. D. (1970a). Effects

of preoptic and spinal cord temperature in control of thermal polypnea. *J. Appl. Physiol.* **28:** 540–542.

Guieu, J. D., and Hardy, J. D. (1970b). Effects of heating and cooling of the spinal cord on preoptic unit activity. *J. Appl. Physiol.* **29:** 675–683.

Haartsen, P. I. (1967). Insulation of floors in livestock buildings. *Farm Mech. Build.* **19:** 25–26.

*Hafez, E. S. E. (1968a). Environmental effects on animal productivity. In *Adaptation of Domestic Animals*, E. S. E. Hafez, Ed. Philadelphia: Lea and Febiger, pp. 74–93.

*Hafez, E. S. E. (1968b). Behavioral adaptation. In *Adaptation of Domestic Animals*, E. S. E. Hafez, Ed. Philadelphia: Lea and Febiger, pp. 202–214.

*Hafez, E. S. E. (1968c). Morphological and anatomical adaptations. In *Adaptation of Domestic Animals*, E. S. E. Hafez, Ed. Philadelphia: Lea and Febiger, p. 72.

Haldane, J. S. (1905). The influence of high air temperatures. *J. Hyg. (Cambridge)* **5:** 494–513.

Haldane, J. S. (1929). Salt depletion by sweating. *Brit. Med. J.* **2:** 469.

Hales, J. R. S., and Findlay, J. D. (1968a). The oxygen cost of thermally-induced hyperventilation in the ox. *Respir. Physiol.* **4:** 353–362.

Hales, J. R. S. and Findlay, J. D. (1968b). Respiration in the ox, normal values and the effects of exposure to hot environments. *Respir. Physiol.* **4:** 333–352.

Hales, J. R. S. and Webster, M. E. D. (1967). Respiratory function during thermal tachypnoea in sheep. *J. Physiol. (London)* **190:** 241–260.

*Hammel, H. T. (1968). Regulation of internal body temperature. *Ann. Rev. Physiol.* **30:** 641–710.

*Hammel, H. T., and Hardy, J. D. (1963). A gradient type of calorimeter for measurement of thermoregulatory responses in the dog. In *Temperature, Its Measurement and Control in Science and Industry*, Vol. III, Pt. 3, J. D. Hardy, Ed. New York: Reinhold, pp. 31–42.

*Hardy, J. D. (1949). Heat transfer. In *Physiology of Heat Regulation and Science of Clothing*, L. H. Newburgh, Ed. Philadelphia: Saunders, pp. 78–108.

*Hardy, J. D. (1961). Physiology of temperature regulation. *Physiol. Rev.* **41:** 521–606.

*Hardy, J. D. (1970). Thermal comfort: skin temperature and physiological thermoregulation. In *Physiological and Behavioral Temperature Regulation*, J. D. Hardy, A. P. Gagge, and J. A. J. Stolwijk, Eds. Springfield, Ill.: Charles C Thomas, Chapter 57, pp. 856–873.

*Hardy, J. D., Stolwijk, J. A. J., and Gagge, A. P. (1971). Man. In *Comparative Physiology of Thermoregulation*, Vol. 2, G. C. Whittow, Ed. New York and London: Academic Press, Chapter 5, pp. 328–378.

Hare, E. H., and Haigh, C. P. (1955). Variations in the iodine activity of the normal human thyroid as measured by the 24 hr ^{131}I uptake. *Clin. Sci.* **4:** 441–449.

*Hart, J. S. (1971). Rodents. In *Comparative Physiology of Thermoregulation*, G. C. Whittow, Ed. New York and London: Academic Press, pp. 2–130.

*Hatch, T. F. (1963). Assessment of heat stress. In *Temperature, Its Measurement and Control in Science and Industry*, Vol. 3, Pt. 3, C. M. Hertzfeld and J. D. Hardy, Eds. New York: Reinhold, pp. 307–318.

Hellmann, K. (1955). Cholinesterase and amine oxidase in the skin: a histochemical investigation. *J. Physiol. (London)* **129:** 454–463.

Hellmann, K., and Collins, K. J. (1957). Thyroid, salivary and Harderian glands in mice exposed to heat. *J. Endocrinol.* **15:** 145–150.

Hellmann, K., Collins, K. J., Gray, C. H., Jones, R. M., Lunnon, J. B., and Weiner, J. S. (1956). The excretion of urinary adrenocortical steroids during heat stress. *J. Endocrinol.* **14:** 209–216.

Hellmann, K., and Weiner, J. S. (1953). Antidiuretic substance in urine following exposure to high temperatures. *J. Appl. Physiol.* **6:** 194–198.

*Hellon, R. (1970). Hypothalamic neurons responding to changes in hypothalamic and ambient temperature. In *Physiological and Behavioral Temperature Regulation*, J. D. Hardy, A. P. Gagge, and J. A. J. Stolwijk, Eds. Springfield, Ill.: Charles C Thomas, pp. 463–471.

Hellon, R. F., and Provins, K. A. (1972). Unit responses in the somatosensory cerebral cortex of the rat following temperature changes in scrotal skin. *J. Physiol. (London)* **222:** 151–152P.

Hemingway, A. (1938). The panting response of normal anaesthetized dogs to measured dosages of diathermy heat. *Am. J. Physiol.* **121:** 747–754.

*Hensel, H. (1963). Electrophysiology of thermosensitive nerve endings. In *Temperature, Its Measurement and Control in Science and Industry*, Vol. 3, Pt. 3, J. D. Hardy, Ed. New York: Reinhold, pp. 191–198.

*Hensel, H. (1973). Temperature receptors in the skin. In *Physiological and Behavioral Temperature Regulation*, J. D. Hardy, A. P. Gagge, and J. A. J. Stolwijk, Eds. Springfield, Ill.: Charles C Thomas, pp. 442–453.

*Hensel, H. (1973). Neural processes in thermoregulation. *Physiol. Rev.* **53:** 948–1017.

Hensel, H., and Witt, I. (1959). Spatial temquantitative study of sensitive cutaneous thermoreceptors with C afferent fibres. *J. Physiol. (London)* **153:** 113–126.

Hensel, H. and Witt, I. (1959). Spatial temperature gradient and thermoreceptor stimulation. *J. Physiol. (London)* **148:** 180–189.

Hermanson, V., and Hartman, F. A. (1945). Protection of adrenalectomised rats against high temperature. *Am. J. Physiol.* **144:** 108–114.

*Hertzman, A. B. (1959). Vasomotor regulation of cutaneous circulation. *Physiol. Rev.* **39:** 280–306.

Hertzman, A. B., Randall, W. C., Peiss, C. N., and Seckendorf, R. (1952). Regional rates of evaporation from the skin at various environmental temperatures. *J. Appl. Physiol.* **5:** 153–161.

Hey, E. N., and Katz, G. (1969). Evaporative water loss in the new-born baby. *J. Physiol. (London)* **200:** 605–619.

Hey, E. N., and Katz, G. (1970). The range of thermal insulation in the tissues of the New-born baby. *J. Physiol. (London)* **207:** 667–681.

Hey, E. N., Katz, G., and O'Connell, B. (1970). The total thermal insulation of the new-born baby. *J. Physiol. (London)* **207:** 683–698.

Hey, E. N., and Mount, L. E. (1966). Temperature control in incubators. *Lancet* **2:** 202–203.

Hey, E. N., and Mount, L. E. (1967). Heat losses from babies in incubators. *Arch. Dis. Child.* **42:** 75–84.

Hill, A. V., and Hill, A. M. (1914). A self-recording calorimeter for large animals. *J. Physiol. (London)* **48:** xiii.

Hoffmann, E., and Shaffner, C. S. (1950). Thyroid weight and function as influenced by environmental temperature. *Poult. Sci.* **29:** 365–376.

Hurley, H. J., and Shelley, W. B. (1954). The role of the myoepithelium of the human apocrine sweat gland. *J. Invest. Derm.* **22:** 143–155.

Hutchinson, J. C. D. (1955). Evaporative cooling in fowls. *J. Agric. Sci. (Cambridge)* **45:** 48–59.

Iggo, A. (1969). Cutaneous thermoreceptors in primates and sub-primates. *J. Physiol. (London)* **200:** 403–430.

Ingram, D. L. (1964a). The effect of environmental temperature on body temperatures respiratory frequency and pulse rate in the young pig. *Res. Vet. Sci.* **5:** 348–356.

Ingram, D. L. (1964b). The effect of environmental temperature on heat loss and thermal insulation in the young pig. *Res. Vet. Sci.* **5:** 357–364.

Ingram, D. L. (1965a). The effect of humidity on temperature regulation and cutaneous water loss in the young pig. *Res. Vet. Sci.* **6:** 9–17.

Ingram, D. L. (1965b). Evaporative cooling in the pig. *Nature (London)* **207:** 415–416.

Ingram, D. L. (1967). Stimulation of cutaneous glands in the pig. *J. Comp. Pathol.* **77:** 93–99.

Ingram, D. L., and Legge, K. F. (1969). The effect of environmental temperature on respiratory ventilation in the pig. *Respir. Physiol.* **8:** 1–12.

Ingram, D. L., and Legge, K. F. (1970a). The thermoregulatory behaviour of young pigs in a natural environment. *Physiol. Behav.* **5:** 981–987.

Ingram, D. L., and Legge, K. F. (1970b). Variations in deep body temperature in the young unrestrained pig over the 24 h period. *J. Physiol. (London)* **210:** 989–998.

Ingram, D. L., and Legge, K. F. (1971). The influence of deep body temperature and skin temperature on peripheral blood flow in the pig. *J. Physiol. (London)* **215:** 693–707.

Ingram, D. L., McLean, J. A., and Whittow, G. C. (1963). The effect of heating the hypothalamus and the skin on the rate of moisture vaporization from the skin of the ox. *J. Physiol. (London)* **169:** 394–403.

Ingram, D. L., and Slebodzinski, A. (1965). Oxygen consumption and thyroid gland activity during adaptation to high ambient temperatures in young pigs. *Res. Vet. Sci.* **6:** 522–530.

Ingram, D. L., and Whittow, G. C. (1962a). The effect of heating the hypothalamus on respiration in the ox (*Bos taurus*). *J. Physiol. (London)* **163:** 200–210.

Ingram, D. L., and Whittow, G. C. (1962b). The effects of variations in respiratory activity and in the skin temperature of the ears on the temperature of the blood in the external jugular vein of the ox (*Bos taurus*). *J. Physiol. (London)* **163:** 211–221.

Ingram, D. L., and Whittow, G. C. (1962c). Changes of arterial blood pressure and heart rate in the ox (*Bos taurus*) with changes of body temperature. *J. Physiol. (London)* **168:** 736–746.

*Irving, L. (1964). Terrestrial animals in cold: Birds and mammals. In *Handbook of Physiology, Section 4: Adaptation to Environment*, D. B. Dill, Ed. Washington, D.C.: American Physiological Society, pp. 361–377.

Itoh, S. (1954). The release of antidiuretic hormone from the posterior pituitary body on exposure to heat. *Japan J. Physiol.* **4:** 185–190.

Jackson, P. C., and Schmidt-Nielsen, K. (1964). Countercurrent heat exchange in respiratory passages. *Proc. Natl. Acad. Sci. U.S.* **51:** 1192–1197.

Jakob, M. (1949). *Heat Transfer.* Vol. I. New York: Wiley.

Jakob, M. (1957). *Heat Transfer.* Vol. II. New York: Wiley.

Jenkinson, D. McE. (1967). On the classification of sweat glands and the question of the existence of an apocrine secretory process. *Brit. Vet. J.* **123:** 311–315.

Jenkinson, D. McE., and Blackburn, P. S. (1967). The distribution of nerves, monoamine oxidase and cholinesterase in the skin of the sheep and goat. *J. Anat.* **101:** 333–341.

Jenkinson, D. McE., Sengupta, B. P., and Blackburn, P. S. (1966). The distribution of nerves, monoamine oxidase and cholinesterase in the skin of cattle. *J. Anat.* **100:** 593–613.

Jessen, C. (1967). Auslösung von Hecheln durch isolierte Wärmung des Rückenmarks an wachen Hund. *Pflügers Arch.* **297:** 53–70.

Johansen, K. (1962). Heat exchange through the muskrat tail. Evidence for vasodilator nerves to the skin. *Acta Physiol. Scand.* **55:** 160–169.

Johnson, H. D., Cheng, C. S., and Ragsdale, A. C. (1958). Influence of rising environmental temperature on the physiological reactions of rabbits and cattle. Univ. Mo. Agric. Exp. Res. Bull. **648.**

Johnson, H. D., and Ragsdale, A. C. (1960). Temperature effects on thyroid I^{131} release rate of dairy calves. *Univ. Mo. Agric. Exp. Res. Bull.* **709.**

Johnson, H. D., Ragsdale, A. C., Berry, I. L., and Shanklin, M. D. (1963). Environmental physiology and shelter engineering—with special reference to domestic animals. LXVI. Temperature-humidity effects including influence of acclimation in feed and water consumption of Holstein cattle. *Univ. Mo. Agric. Exp. Res. Bull.* **846:** 43.

Johnson, H. D., Ward, M. W., and Kibler, H. H. (1966). Heat and aging effects of thyroid function of male rats. *J. Appl. Physiol.* **21:** 689–694.

Joyce, J. P., Blaxter, K. L., and Park, C. (1966). The effect of natural out-door environments on the energy requirements of sheep. *Res. Vet. Sci.* **7:** 342–359.

Kahl, M. P. (1963). Thermoregulation in the wood stork, with special references to the role of the legs. *Physiol. Zool.* **36:** 141–151.

Keeton, R. W. (1924). The peripheral water loss in rabbits as a factor in heat regulation. *Am J. Physiol.* **69:** 307–317.

Kelly, C. F., Bond, T. E., and Heitman, H., Jr. (1963). Direct "air" calorimetry for livestock. *Trans. Am. Soc. Agric. Eng.* **6:** 126–128.

*Kerslake, D. McK. (1972). *The Stress of Hot Environments.* London: Cambridge University Press.

*Kerslake, D. McK., and Brebner, D. F. (1970). Maximum sweating at rest. In *Physiological and Behavioral Temperature Regulation*, J. D. Hardy, A. P. Gagge, and J. A. J. Stolwijk, Eds. Springfield, Ill.: Charles C Thomas, pp. 139–151.

*King, J. R., and Farner, D. S. (1964). Terrestrial animals in humid heat: birds. In *Handbook of Physiology, Section 4: Adaptation to Environment*, D. B. Dill, Ed. Washington, D.C.: American Physiological Society, pp. 603–624.

*Kirmiz, J. P. (1962). *Adaptation to Desert Environment.* London: Butterworths.

*Kleiber, M. (1961). *The Fire of Life.* New York: Wiley.

Kleiber, M., and Regan, W. (1933). Influence of temperature on respiration of cows. *Proc. Soc. Exp. Biol. Med.* **33:** 10–14.

*Klussman, F. W., and Pierau, F. K. (1972). Extrahypothalamic deep body thermosensitivity. In *Essays on Temperature Regulation*, J. Bligh and R. E. Moore, Eds. Amsterdam and London: North Holland.

Kosaka, M., Simon, E., Thauer, R., and Wather, O. E. (1969). Effect of thermal stimulation of spinal cord on respiratory and cortical activity. *Am. J. Physiol.* **217:** 858–864.

Kullman, R., Schönung, W., and Simon, E. (1970). Antagonistic changes of blood flow and sympathetic activity in different vascular beds following central stimulation. I. Blood flow in skin muscle and intestine during spinal cord heating and cooling in anesthetized dogs. *Pflügers Arch.* **319:** 146–161.

*Kuno, Y. (1956). *The Physiology of Human Perspiration*, 2nd ed. London: Churchill.

*Landgren, S. (1970). Projections from thermoreceptors into the somatosensory system of the cat's brain. In *Physiological and Behavioral Temperature Regulation*, J. D. Hardy, A. P. Gagge, and J. A. J. Stolwijk, Eds. Springfield, Ill.: Charles C Thomas.

Lasiewski, R. C., Acosta, A. L., and Bernstein, M. H. (1966). Evaporative water loss in birds. 1. Characteristics of the open-flow method of determination, and their relation to estimates of thermoregulatory ability. *Comp. Biochem. Physiol.* **19:** 459–470.

Lee, D. H. K., Robinson, K., and Hines, H. J. G. (1941). Reactions of the rabbit to hot atmospheres. *Proc. Roy. Soc. (Queensland)* **53:** 129–158.

*Leithead, C. S., and Lind, A. R. (1964). *Heat Stress and Heat Disorders.* London: Cassell.

Lewis, H. E., Foster, A. R., Mullan, B. J., Cox, R. N., and Clark, R. P. (1969). Aerodynamics of the human microenvironment. *Lancet* **1:** 1273–1277.

Lewis, T., and Pickering, G. W. (1931). Vasodilatation in the limbs in response to warming the body with evidence for sympathetic vasodilator nerves in man. *Heart* **16:** 33–51.

*Lind, A. R. (1963). Tolerable limits for prolonged and intermittent exposures to heat. In *Temperature, Its Measurement and Control in Science and Industry*, Vol. 3, Pt. 3, Hardy, J. D., Ed. New York: Reinhold, pp. 337–345.

Lipton, J. M. (1971). Behavioral temperature regulation in the rat: effect of thermal stimulation of the medulla. *J. Physiol. (Paris)* **63:** 325–328.

*Louw, G. N. (1972). The role of advective fog in the water economy of certain Namib Desert animals. In *Comparative Physiology of Desert Animals*, G. M. O. Maloiy, Ed. London: Academic Press, pp. 297–314.

Lusk, G. (1928). *The Elements of the Science of Nutrition*, 4th ed. Philadelphia: Saunders.

*Macfarlane, W. V. (1963). Endocrine functions in hot environments. In: *Environmental Physiology and Psychology in Arid Conditions, Reviews of Research*, Vol. 22. Paris: Unesco, pp. 153–222.

*Macfarlane, W. V. (1964). Terrestrial animals in dry heat: ungulates. In *Handbook of Physiology, Section 4: Adaptation to Environment*, D. B. Dill, Ed. Washington, D.C.: American Physiological Society, pp. 509–539.

*Macfarlane, W. V. (1968a). Adaptation of ruminants to tropics and deserts. In *Adaptation of Domestic Animals*, E. S. E. Hafez, Ed. Philadelphia: Lea and Febiger, pp. 164–182.

*Macfarlane, W. V. (1968b). Comparative functions of ruminants in hot environments. In *Adaptation of Domestic Animals*, E. S. E. Hafez, Ed. Philadelphia: Lea and Febiger, pp. 264–276.

Macfarlane, W. V., Pennycuik, P. R., Yeates, N. T. M., and Thrift, E. (1959). Reproduction in hot environments. In *Recent Progress in the Endocrinology of Reproduction*. C. W. Lloyd, Ed. New York: Academic Press, pp. 81–95.

Macfarlane, W. V. and Robinson, K. W. (1957). Seasonal changes in plasma antidiuretic activity produced by a standard heat stimulus. *J. Physiol. (London)* **135:** 1–11.

MacGregor, R. G. S., and Loh, G. L. (1941). The influence of a tropical environment upon the basal metabolism, pulse rate and blood pressure in Europeans. *J. Physiol. (London)* **99:** 496–509.

Macpherson, R. K. (1960). Physiological responses to hot environments. Med. Res. Co. Spec. Rep. Ser. 298. London: H.M.S.O.

Magoun, H. W., Harrison, F., Brobeck, J. R., and Ranson, S. W. (1938). Activation of heat loss mechanisms by local heating of the brain. *J. Neurophysiol.* **1:** 101–114.

Mansfeld, A. (1946). Thermothyrin A and B: temperature-regulating hormones of the thyroid. *Nature (London)* **157:** 491.

Mather, G. W., Nahas, G. G., and Hemmingway, A. (1953). Temperature changes of pulmonary blood during exposure to cold. *Am. J. Physiol.* **173:** 390–393.

McArdle, B., Dunham, W., Holling, H. E., Ladel, W. S. S., Scott, J. W., Thomson, M. L., and Weiner, J. S. (1947). The prediction of the physiological effects of warm and hot environments. Rept. No. RNP 47/391, Med. Res. Council, London.

McCutchan, J. W., and Taylor, C. L. (1951). Respiratory heat exchange with varying temperature and humidity of inspired air. *J. Appl. Physiol.* **4:** 121–135.

*McDowell, R. E. (1972). *Improvement of Livestock Production in Warm Climates.* San Francisco: W. H. Freeman and Co.

McGuire, J. H. (1953). Heat transfer by radiation. D.S.I.R. Fire Research Special Rept. No. 2. London: H.M.S.O.

McLean, J. A. (1963a). Measurement of cutaneous moisture vaporization from cattle by ventilated capsules. *J. Physiol. (London)* **167:** 417–426.

McLean, J. A. (1963b). The partition of insensible losses of body weight and heat from cattle under various climatic conditions. *J. Physiol. (London)* **167:** 427–447.

*McWhinnie, M. A. (1967). The heat responses of invertebrates (exclusive of insects). In *Thermobiology*, A. H. Rose, Ed. London: Academic Press, pp. 353–373.

Mendelsohn, E. (1964). *The Development of the Theory of Animal Heat.* Cambridge, Mass.: Harvard University Press.

Meyer, H. H. (1913). Theorie des Fiebers und seine Behandlung. *Zentr. Inn. Med.* **6:** 385–386.

*Minard, D. (1970). Body heat content. In *Physiological and Behavioral Temperature Regulation*, J. D. Hardy, A. P. Gagge, and J. A. J. Stolwijk, Eds. Springfield, Ill.: Charles C Thomas, pp. 345–357.

*Mitchell, D. (1970). Measurement of the thermal emissivity of human skin *in vivo*. In *Physiological and Behavioral Temperature Regulation*, J. D. Hardy, A. P. Gagge, and J. A. J. Stolwijk, Eds. Springfield, Ill.: Charles C Thomas, pp. 25–33.

*Mitchell, D. (1974). Convective heat transfer from man and other animals. In *Heat Loss from Animals and Man: Assessment and Control*, J. L. Monteith and L. E. Mount, Eds. London: Butterworths, pp. 59–76.

*Mitchell, D., Atkins, A. R., and Wyndham, C. H. (1972). Mathematical and physical models of thermoregulation. In *Essays on Temperature Regulation*, J. Bligh and R. E. Moore, Eds. Amsterdam and London: North Holland, pp. 37–54.

Montagna, W. (1956). *The Structure and Function of Skin.* New York: Academic Press.

*Monteith, J. L. (1973). *Principles of Environmental Physics.* London: Edward Arnold.

*Monteith, J. L. (1974). Specification of the

environment in relation to heat loss. In *Heat Loss from Animals and Man: Assessment and Control*, J. L. Monteith and L. E. Mount, Eds. London: Butterworths, pp. 1–17.

*Moule, G. R. (1968). World distribution of domestic animals. In *Adaptation of Domestic Animals*, E. S. E. Hafez, Ed. Philadelphia: Lea and Febiger, pp. 18–33.

Moule, G. R., and Waites, G. M. H. (1963). Seminal degeneration in the ram and its relation to the temperature of the scrotum. *J. Reprod. Fert.* **5:** 433–446.

Mount, L. E. (1963). The environmental temperature preferred by the young pig. *Nature London* **199:** 1212–1213.

Mount, L. E. (1964a). Radiant and convective heat loss from the new-born pig. *J. Physiol. (London)* **173:** 96–113.

Mount, L. E. (1964b). The tissue and air components of thermal insulation in the new-born pig. *J. Physiol. (London)* **170:** 286–295.

Mount, L. E. (1966). Thermal and metabolic comparisons between the new-born pig and human infant. In *Swine in Biomedical Research*, L. K. Bustad and R. O. McClellan, Eds. Seattle: Batelle Memorial Institute, pp. 501–509.

*Mount, L. E. (1968a). *The Climatic Physiology of the Pig*. London: Edward Arnold.

*Mount, L. E. (1968b). Adaptation of swine. In *Adaptation of Domestic Animals*, E. S. E. Hafez, Ed. Philadelphia: Lea and Febiger, p. 285.

*Mount, L. E. (1974). Thermal neutrality. In *Heat Loss from Animals and Man: Assessment and Control*, J. L. Monteith and L. E. Mount, Eds. London: Butterworths.

Mount, L. E., and Ingram, D. L. (1964). The effects of ambient temperature and air movement on localized sensible heat loss from the pig. *Res. Vet. Sci.* **6:** 84–91.

Mount, L. E., and Stephens, D. B. (1970). The relation between body size and maximum and minimum metabolic rates in the new-born pig. *J. Physiol. (London)* **207:** 417–427.

Mueller, W. J. (1966). Effect of rapid temperature changes on acid-base balance and shell quality. *Poult. Sci.* **45:** 1109.

Mugass, J. N. and Templeton, J. R. (1970).

Thermoregulation in the red-breasted nuthatch. *Condor* **72:** 125–132.

*Murgatroyd, D., and Hardy, J. D. (1970). Central and peripheral temperatures in behavioral thermoregulation of the rat. In *Physiological and Behavioral Temperature Regulation*, J. D. Hardy, A. P. Gagge, and J. A. J. Stolwijk, Eds. Springfield, Ill.: Charles C Thomas, Chapter 58, pp. 874–891.

Murrish, D. E., and Schmidt-Nielsen, K. (1970). Exhaled air temperature and water conservation in lizards. *Resp. Physiol.* **10:** 151–158.

*Myers, R. D. (1971). Primates. In *Comparative Physiology of Thermoregulation*, Vol. 2, G. C. Whittow, Ed. New York: Academic Press, Chapter 4, pp. 283–323.

Myers, R. D., and Yaksh, T. L. (1971). Thermoregulation around a new "set point" established in the monkey by altering the ratio of sodium to calcium ions within the hypothalamus. *J. Physiol. (London)* **218:** 609–633.

Myhre, K., and Hammel, T. H. (1969). Behavioral regulation of internal temperature inf the lizard, *Tiliqua scincoides. Am. J. Physiol.* **217:** 1490–1495.

Nakayama, T., Eisenman, J. S., and Hardy, J. D. (1961). Single unit activity of anterior hypothalamus during local heating. *Science* **134:** 560–561.

Nakayama, T., and Hardy, J. D. (1969). Unit response in the rabbit's brain stem to changes in brain and cutaneous temperature. *J. Appl. Physiol.* **27:** 848–857.

O'Connor, W. R. (1962). Renal function. London: Arnold.

*Ogawa, T. (1973). Local determinants of sweat gland activity. In *Advances in Climatic Physiology*, S. Itoh, K. Ogata, and H. Yoshimura, Eds. Tokyo: Igaku Shoin; Berlin, Heidelberg, and New York: Springer-Verlag, pp. 93–108.

*Ohara, K. (1972). Salt concentration in sweat and heat adaptability. In *Advances in Climatic Physiology*, S. Itoh, K. Ogota, and H. Yoshimura, Eds. Tokyo: Igaku Shoin; Berlin, Heidelberg, and New York: Springer-Verlag, pp. 122–133.

Otis, A. B. (1954). The work of breathing. *Physiol. Rev.* **34:** 449–458.

Otis, A. B., Fenn, W. O., and Rahn, H. (1950). Mechanics of breathing in man. *J. Appl. Physiol.* **2**: 592–607.

Pan, Y. S. (1963). Quantitative and morphological variation of sweat glands, skin thickness and skin shrinkage over various body regions of Sahiwal Zebu and Jersey cattle. *Aust. J. Agric. Res.* **3**: 424–437.

*Pepler, R. D. (1963). Performance and well-being in heat. In *Temperature, Its Measurement and Control in Science and Industry*, Pt. 3, Vol. 3, J. D. Hardy, Ed. New York: Reinhold, pp. 319–336.

Peter, J., and Wyndham, C. H. (1966). Activity of the human eccrine sweat gland during exercise in a hot humid environment before and after acclimatization. *J. Physiol. (London)* **187**: 583–594.

Phillips, R. W., and McKenzie, F. F. (1934). The thermoregulatory function and mechanism of the scrotum. *Res. Bull. Mo. Agric. Exp. Stn.* **217**: 1–73.

Pickering, G. W., and Hess, W. (1933). Vasodilatation in the hands and feet in response to warming the body. *Clin. Sci.* **1**: 213–223.

Pitesky, I., and Last, J. H. (1951). Effects of seasonal heat stress on glomerular and tubular functions in the dog. *Am. J. Physiol.* **164**: 497–501.

Prouty, L. R., Barrett, M. J., and Hardy, J. D. (1949). A simple calorimeter for the simultaneous determination of heat loss and heat production in animals. *Rev. Sci. Instrum.* **20**: 357–363.

Provins, K. A., Hellon, R. F., Bell, C. R., and Hirons, R. W. (1962). Tolerance to heat of subjects in sedentary work. *Ergonomics* **5**: 93–97.

Pullar, J. D. (1958). Direct calorimetry of animals by the gradient layer principle. *First Symposium on Energy Metabolism.* Rome: European Association for Animal Production.

Radigan, L. R., and Robinson, S. (1949). Effects of environmental heat stress and exercise on renal blood flow and filtration rate. *J. Appl. Physiol.* **2**: 185–191.

Ragsdale, A. C., Thompson, H. J., Worstell, D. M., and Brody, S. (1951). Environmental Physiology—with special reference to domestic animals. XII. Influence of increasing of temperature, 40° to 105°F on milk production in Brown Swiss cows, and on feed and water consumption and body weight in Brown Swiss and Brahman cows and heifers. *Univ. Mo. Agric. Exp. Stn. Res. Bull.* **471**: 24.

Ragsdale, A. C., Thompson, H. J., Worstell, D. M., and Brody, S. (1953). Environmental physiology and shelter engineering—with special reference to domestic animals. XXI. The effect of humidity on milk production and composition, feed and water consumption, and body weight in cattle. *Univ. Mo. Agric. Exp. Stn. Res. Bull.* **521**: 24.

Rand, R. P., Burtin, A. C., and Ing. T. (1965). The tail of the rat, in temperature regulation and acclimatization. *Can. J. Physiol. Pharmacol.* **43**: 257–267.

*Randall, W. C. (1963). Sweating and its neural control. In *Temperature, its Measurement and Control in Science and Industry*, C. M. Hertzfeld and J. D. Hardy, Eds. Vol. 3, Pt. 3, London and New York: Reinhold, pp. 275–286.

Randall, W. C., and Hertzman, A. B. (1953). Dermatomal recruitment of sweating. *J. Appl. Physiol.* **5**: 399–409.

Ranson, S. W., and Ingram, W. R. (1935). Hypothalamus and regulation of body temperature. *Proc. Soc. Exp. Biol. Med.* **32**: 1439–1441.

Ranson, S. W., and Magoun, H. W. (1939). The hypothalamus. *Ergeb. Physiol. Biol. Chem. Exp. Pharmakol.* **41**: 56–163.

*Rapp, G. M. (1970). Convective mass transfer and the coefficient of evaporative heat loss from human skin. In *Physiological and Behavioral Temperature Regulation*, J. D. Hardy, A. P. Gagge, and J. A. J. Stolwijk, Eds. Springfield, Ill.: Charles C Thomas, pp. 55–80.

Regal, P. J. (1971). Long term studies with operant conditioning techniques of temperature regulation patterns in reptiles. *J. Physiol. (Paris)* **63**: 403–406.

Reignault, V., and Reiset, J. (1849). Recherches chimiques sur la respiration des animaux. *Ann. Chim. Phys. Ser. 3* **26**: 299–519.

Richards, J. B., and Egdahl, R. H. (1956). Effect of acute hyperthermia on adrenal 17-hydroxycorticosteroid secretion in dogs. *Am. J. Physiol.* **186**: 435–439.

*Richards, S. A. (1970). The biology and comparative physiology of thermal panting. *Biol. Rev.* **45:** 223–264.

*Richards, S. A. (1974). Aspects of physical thermoregulation in the fowl. In *Heat Loss from Animals and Man: Assessment and Control*, J. L. Monteith and L. E. Mount, Eds. London: Butterworths, pp. 255–275.

Richet, C. (1889). *La Chaleur Animale.* Bibliothèque Scientifique International, Paris: Felix Alcan.

Rick, R. F., Hardy, M. H., Lee, D. K. H., and Carter, H. B. (1950). The effect of the dietary plane upon reactions of two breeds of sheep during short exposures to hot environments. *Aust. J. Agric. Res.* **1:** 217–230.

Robertshaw, D. (1968). The pattern and control of sweating in the sheep and the goat. *J. Physiol London* **198:** 531–539.

Robertshaw, D., and Taylor, C. R. (1969). Sweat gland function of the donkey *(Equus asinus). J. Physiol. (London)* **205:** 79–89.

Robinson, K., and Lee, D. H. K. (1941). Reactions of the cat to hot atmospheres. *Proc. Roy. Soc. (Queensland)* **53:** 159–170.

*Robinson, S. (1949). Physiological adjustments to heat. In *Physiology of Heat Regulation and the Science of Clothing*, L. H. Newburgh, Ed. Philadelphia: Saunders, pp. 193–239.

*Robinson, S. (1963). Circulatory adjustments of men in hot environments. In *Temperature, its Measurement and Control in Science and Industry*, Vol. 3, Pt. 3, C. M. Hertzfeld and J. D. Hardy, Eds. New York: Reinhold, pp. 287–297.

*Robinson, S., and Robinson, A. H. (1954). Chemical composition of sweat. *Physiol. Rev.* **34:** 202–220.

Robinson, S., Turrell, E. S., and Gerking, S. D. (1945). Physiologically equivalent conditions of air temperature and humidity. *Am. J. Physiol.* **143:** 21–32.

Rothman, S. (1954). *Physiology and Biochemistry of the Skin.* Chicago: University of Chicago Press.

Rozin, P. N., and Mayer, J. (1961). Thermal reinforcement and thermoregulatory behavior in the goldfish, *Carassius auratus. Science* **134:** 942–943.

Rubner, M. (1894). Die Quelle der thierischen Wärme. *Biologie* **30:** 73–142.

*Salt, G. W. (1964). Respiratory evaporation in birds. *Biol. Rev.* **39:** 113–136.

Salt, G. W., and Zeuthen, E. (1960). The respiratory system. In *Biology and Comparative Physiology of Birds*, Vol. 1, A. J. Marshall, Ed. New York and London: Academic Press, Chapter 10, 363–404.

Satinoff, E. (1964). Behavioural thermoregulation in response to local cooling of rat brain. *Am. J. Physiol.* **206:** 1389–1394.

Sayers, G., and Sayers, M. A. (1947). Regulation of pituitary adrenocorticotrophic activity during the response of the rat to acute stress. *Endocrinology* **40:** 265–273.

Schmidt, I. G., and Schmidt, L. H. (1938). Variations in the structure of adrenals and thyroids produced by thyroxine and high environmental temperatures. *Endocrinology* **23:** 559–565.

*Schmidt-Nielsen, K. (1954). Heat regulation in small and large desert mammals. In *Biology of Deserts*, J. L. Cloudsley-Thompson, Ed. London: Institute of Biology, pp. 182–187.

*Schmidt-Nielsen, K. (1963). Heat conservation in countercurrent systems. In *Temperature, Its Measurement and Control in Science and Industry*, J. D. Hardy, Ed. New York: Reinhold, pp. 143–148.

*Schmidt-Nielsen, K. (1964). *Desert Animals; Physiological Problems of Heat and Water.* London: Oxford University Press.

Schmidt-Nielsen, K., Bretz, W. L., and Taylor, C. R. (1970). Panting in dogs: unidirectional flow over evaporative surfaces. *Science* **169:** 1102–1104.

Schmidt-Nielsen, K., Hainsworth, F. R., and Murrish, D. E. (1969). Cooling of expired air by counter-current exchange. *Fed. Proc.* **28:** 459.

Schmidt-Nielsen, K., Hainsworth, F. R., and Murrish, D. E. (1970). Counter-current heat exchange in the respiratory passages: Effect on water and heat balance. *Resp. Physiol.* **9:** 263–276.

Schmidt-Nielsen, K., Taylor, C. R., and Shkolnik, A. (1971). Desert snails: Problems of heat, water and food. *J. Exp. Biol.* **55:** 385–398.

*Schmidt-Nielsen, K., Taylor, C. R., and Shkolnik, A. (1972). Desert snails: Problems of survival. In *Comparative Physiology of Desert Animals*, G. M. O. Maloiy, Ed. London: Academic Press, pp. 1–13.

Scholander, P. F., and Krog, J. (1957). Countercurrent heat exchange and vascular bundles in sloths. *J. Appl. Physiol.* **10:** 405–411.

Schwartz, I. L., Thaysen, J. H., and Dole, V. P. (1953). Urea excretion in human sweat as a tracer for movement of water within the secreting gland. *J. Exp. Med.* **97:** 429–437.

Scott, J. C., Bazett, H. C., and Mackie, G. C. (1940). Climatic effects on cardiac output and the circulation in man. *Am. J. Physiol.* **129:** 102–122.

Seath, D. M., and Millar, G. D. (1946). Effect of warm weather on grazing performance of milking cows. *J. Dairy Sci.* **29:** 199–206.

Seckendorff, R., and Randall, W. C. (1961). Thermal reflex sweating in normal and paraplegic man. *J. Appl. Physiol.* **16:** 796–800.

Shanklin, M. D., and Stewart, R. E. (1958). Relief of thermally induced stress in dairy cattle by radiation cooling. *Univ. Mo. Agric. Exp. Stn. Res. Bull.* **670:** 31.

Shelley, W. B., and Hurley, H. J. (1952). Methods of exploring human apocrine gland physiology. *Arch. Derm. Syph.* **66:** 156–161, 172–179.

Shelley, W. B., and Hurley, H. J. (1953). The physiology of the human axillary apocrine sweat gland. *J. Invest. Derm.* **20:** 285–295.

Shelley, W. B., and Mescon, H. (1952). Histochemical demonstration of secretory activity in human eccrine sweat glands. *J. Invest. Derm.* **18:** 289–301.

*Shepherd, J. T., and Webb-Peploe, M. M. (1970). Cardiac output and blood flow distribution during work in heat. In *Physiological and Behavioral Temperature Regulation*, J. D. Hardy, A. P. Gagge, and J. A. J. Stolwijk, Eds. Springfield, Ill.: Charles C Thomas, pp. 237–253.

*Sibbons, J. L. H. (1970). Coefficients of evaporative heat transfer. In *Physiological and Behavioral Temperature Regulation*, J. D. Hardy, A. P. Gagge, and J. A. J. Stolwijk, Eds. Springfield, Ill.: Charles C Thomas, pp. 108–138.

*Siegel, H. S. (1968). Adaptation of poultry.

In *Adaptation of Domestic Animals*, E. S. E. Hafez, Ed. Philadelphia: Lea and Febiger, pp. 292–309.

Simon, E. (1968). Spinal mechanisms of temperature regulation. *Intl. Physiol. Congr. 24*, Washington, D.C., pp. 289–290.

Simon, E., and Iriki, M. (1971). Sensory transmission of spinal heat and cold sensitivity in ascending spinal neurons. *Pflügers Arch. Ges. Physiol.* **328:** 103–120.

*Siple, P. A. (1949). Clothing and climate. In *Physiology of Heat Regulation and the Science of Clothing*, L. H. Newburgh, Ed. Philadelphia: Saunders, pp. 389–442.

Smith, J. H., Robinson, S., and Pearcy, M. (1952). Renal responses to exercise, heat and dehydration. *J. Appl. Physiol.* **4:** 659–665.

Snell, E. S. (1954). Relationship between vasomotor response in the hand and heat changes in the body induced by intravenous infusions of hot or cold saline. *J. Physiol. (London)* **125:** 361–372.

Snellen, J. W. (1967). Mean body temperature and the control of thermal sweating. *Acta Physiol. Pharmacol. Néerl.* **14:** 99–174.

Spealman, C. R. (1945). Effect of ambient air temperature and of hand temperature on blood flow in hands. *Am. J. Physiol.* **145:** 218–222.

*Sperelakis, N. (1970). Temperature effects on excitable cells. In *Physiological and Behavioral Temperature Regulation*, J. D. Hardy, A. P. Gagge, and J. A. J. Stolwijk, Eds. Springfield, Ill.: Charles C Thomas, pp. 408–441.

Steen, I., and Steen, J. B. (1965). Thermoregulatory importance of the beaver's tail. *Comp. Biochem. Physiol.* **15:** 267–270.

Stein, G., Sturkie, P. D., and Whittow, G. C. (1964). Changes in the cardiac output, blood pressure and heart rate of the chicken during hypothermia. *J. Physiol. (London)* **170:** 61–62P.

Stitt, J. T., Adair, E. R., Nadel, E. R., and Stolwijk, J. A. J. (1971). The relation between behavior and physiology in the thermoregulatory response of the squirrel monkey. *J. Physiol. (Paris)* **63:** 424–427.

Stower, W. J. and Griffiths, J. F. (1966). The body temperature of the desert locust (*Schistocerca gregaria*). *Entomol. Exp. Appl.* **9:** 127–178.

Ström, G. (1950). The influence of local thermal stimulation of the hypothalamus of the cat on cutaneous blood flow and respiratory rate. *Acta Physiol. Scand.* **20:** Suppl. 70, 47–76.

Strømme, S. B., Myhre, K., and Hammel, H. T. (1971). Forebrain temperature activates behavioral thermoregulatory response in arctic sculpins. *J. Physiol. (Paris)* **63:** 433–435.

*Strydom, N. B., and Wyndham, C. H. (1963). Natural state of heat acclimatization of different ethnic groups. *Fed. Proc.* **22:** 801–809.

Taylor, C. R. (1966). The vascularity and possible thermoregulatory function of the horns in goats. *Physiol. Zool.* **39:** 127–139.

Taylor, C. R. (1970). Strategies of temperature regulation: effect on evaporation in East African ungulates. *Am. J. Physiol.* **219:** 1131–1135.

*Taylor, C. R. (1972). The desert gazelle: a paradox resolved. In *Comparative Physiology of Desert Animals*, G. M. O. Maloiy, Ed. London: Academic Press, pp. 215–227.

Templeton, J. R. (1960). Respiration and water loss at higher temperatures in the desert iguana, *Dipsosaurus dorsalis*. *Physiol. Zool.* **33:** 136–145.

*Templeton, J. R. (1970). Reptiles. In *Comparative Physiology of Thermoregulation*, Vol. 1, G. C. Whittow, Ed. New York: Academic Press, pp. 167–221.

Templeton, J. R., and Dawson, W. R. (1963). Respiration in the lizard, *Crotalphytus collaris*. *Physiol. Zool.* **36:** 104–121.

*Thauer, R. (1965). Circulatory adjustments to climatic requirements. In *Handbook of Physiology—Circulation*, Sec. 2, Vol. III, D. B. Dill, Ed. Washington, D.C.: American Physiological Society, pp. 1921–1966.

*Thauer, R. (1970). Thermosensitivity of the spinal cord. In *Physiological and Behavioral Temperature Regulation*, J. D. Hardy, A. P. Gagge, and J. A. J. Stolwijk, Eds. Springfield, Ill.: Charles C Thomas, pp. 472–492.

Tucker, V. A. (1962). Diurnal torpidity in the California pocket mouse. *Science* **136:** 380–381.

Van Heyringen, R. E., and Weiner, J. S. (1952). A comparison of arm-bag sweat and body sweat. *J. Physiol. (London)* **116:** 395–403.

Waites, G. M. H. (1962). The effect of heating the scrotum of the ram on respiration and body temperature. *Quart. J. Exp. Physiol.* **47:** 314–323.

*Waites, G. M. H. (1970). Temperature regulation of the testis. In *The Testis* Vol. 1. Johnson, Gromes, and Vandemark, Eds. New York: Academic Press, pp. 241–279.

Waites, G. M. H., and Moule, G. R. (1961). Relation of vascular heat exchange to temperature regulation in the testis of the ram. *J. Reprod. Fert.* **2:** 213–224.

Waites, G. M. H. and Setchell, B. P. (1964). Effect of local heating on blood flow and metabolism in the testis of the conscious ram. *J. Reprod. Fert.* **8:** 339–349.

Waites, G. M. H., and Voglmayr, J. K. (1963). The functional activity and control of the apocrine sweat glands of the scrotum of the ram. *Aust. J. Agric. Res.* **6:** 839–851.

Walker, J. E. C., Wells, R. E., Jr., and Merrill, E. W. (1961). Heat and water exchange in the respiratory tract. *Am. J. Med.* **30:** 259–267.

Walther, O. E., Simon, E., and Jessen, C. (1971). Thermoregulatory adjustments of skin blood flow in chronically spinalized dogs. *Pflügers Arch. Ges. Physiol.* **322:** 323–335.

Warburg, M. R. (1972). Water economy and thermal balance of Israeli and Australian amphibia from xeric habitats. *Symp. Zool. Soc. Lond.* **31:** 79–111.

Webb-Peploe, M. M., and Shepherd, J. T. (1968). Response of dog's cutaneous veins to local and central temperature changes. *Circ. Res.* **23:** 693–699.

*Weiner, J. S., and Hellman, K. (1960). The sweat glands. *Biol. Rev.* **35:** 141–186.

Weiner, J. S., and van Heyningen, R. E. (1952). Salt losses of men working in hot environments. *Brit. J. Indust. Med.* **9:** 56–64.

Weiss, B., and Laties, V. G. (1961). Behavioral thermoregulation. *Science* **133:** 1338–1344.

Wezler, K., and Thauer, R. (1943). Der Kreislauf im Dienste der Wärmeregulation. *Z. Ges Exp. Med.* **112:** 345–379.

White, F. N. (1973). Temperature and the Galapagos marine iguana: insight into reptilian thermoregulation. *Comp. Biochem. Physiol.* **45A:** 503–513.

Whittow, G. C. (1962). The significance of the extremities of the ox (*Bos taurus*) in thermoregulation. *J. Agric. Sci. (Cambridge)* **58:** 109–120.

Whittow, G. C. (1965). The effect of hyperthermia on the systemic and pulmonary circulation of the ox (*Bos taurus*). *Quart. J. Exp. Physiol.* **50:** 300–311.

Whittow, G. C. (1968). Cardiovascular response to localized heating of the anterior hypothalamus. *J. Physiol. (London)* **198:** 541–548.

Whittow, G. C., and Findlay, J. D. (1968). Oxygen cost of thermal panting. *Am. J. Physiol.* **214:** 94–99.

Whittow, G. C., Sturkie, P. D., and Stein, G. (1964). Cardiovascular changes associated with thermal polypnea in the chicken. *Am. J. Physiol.* **207:** 1349–1353.

Wigglesworth, V. B. (1965). *The Principles of Insect Physiology*. London: Methuen.

Willcroft, D. C., and Anderson, J. D. (1960). Effect of acclimatization on the preferred body temperature of the lizard, *Sceloporus accidentalis*. *Science* **131:** 610–611.

Wilson, W. O., Hillerman, J. P., and Edwards, W. H. (1952). The relation of high environmental temperatures to feather and skin temperatures of laying pullets. *Poult. Sci.* **31:** 843–846.

Winslow, C.-E. A., Gagge, A. P., and Herrington, L. P. (1940). Heat exchange and regulation in radiant environments above and below air temperature. *Am. J. Physiol.* **131:** 79–92.

Wit, A., and Wang, S. C. (1968). Temperature-sensitive neurons in preoptic/anterior hypothalamic region: effects of increasing ambient temperature. *Amer. J. Physiol.* **215:** 1151–1159.

Worstell, D. M., and Brody, S. (1953). Environmental physiology and shelter engineering—with special reference to domestic animals. XX. Comparative physiological reactions of European and Indian cattle to changing temperature. *Univ. Mo. Agric. Exp. Stn. Bull.* **515:** 42.

Wünnenberg, W., and Brück, K. (1968). Single unit activity evoked by thermal stimulation of the cervical cord in the guinea pig. *Nature (London)* **218:** 1268–1269.

*Wyndham, C. H. (1970). The problem of heat intolerance in man. In *Physiological and Behavioral Temperature Regulation*, J. D. Hardy, A. P. Gagge, and J. A. J. Stolwijk, Eds. Springfield, Ill.: Charles C Thomas, pp. 324–341.

Wyndham, C. H., Morrison, J. F., and Williams, C. G. (1965). Heat reactions of male and female Caucasians. *J. Appl. Physiol.* **20:** 357–364.

Wyndham, C. H., Strydom, N. B., Morrison, J. F., du Toit, F. D., and Kraan, J. G. (1954). Responses of unacclimatized men under stress of heat and work. *J. Appl. Physiol.* **6:** 681–686.

*Yoshimura, H. (1960). Acclimatization to heat and cold. In *Essential Problems in Climatic Physiology*. H. Yoshimura, K. Ogata, and S. Itoh, Eds. Kyoto: Nankodo.

*Yousef, M. K., Hahn, L., and Johnson, H. D. (1968). Adaptation of cattle. In *Adaptation of Domestic Animals*, E. S. E. Hafez, Ed. Philadelphia: Lea and Febiger, pp. 233–245.

Index